UNTANGLE
YOUR ANXIETY

*A Guide to Overcoming an Anxiety Disorder
by Two People Who Have Been Through It*

JOSHUA FLETCHER & DEAN STOTT

We dedicate this book to all the resilient people who tolerate anxiety every day, thanks to their courage and stoicism.

Table of Contents

Chapter 1

If You Are Anxious, Start Here

Featured Artist: @simplysophiedesigns

Firstly, well done for picking up this book.

We know that constant worry can make it really difficult to concentrate, plus reading whilst anxious is exhausting, so let's get straight to the point.

If you're currently anxious, then let us make this very clear: *this is ok.* Being anxious does not mean something bad is about to happen, nor does it mean that those scary thoughts are any more likely to happen. How you feel does not mean you are about to lose control, lose your mind, collapse, or fall under the weight of your worries. It does not mean that catastrophe you have been ruminating about is any more real than it was this morning. This is what anxiety does; anxiety likes to show you a video reel of all the unpleasant disasters that can occur as a result of this deeply unpleasant feeling.

Let's look at things with a bit more rationality: being excessively anxious means that your mind and body are trying to *protect* you from danger. However, if you are reading this book, then the likelihood is that you are not in any danger at all, but the anxious mind likes to make sure you are safe (just in case you *are* in danger!). The discomfort you are feeling is from your very healthy nervous system activating the fight-or-flight response, which means you are currently feeling the 'on-edge' effects of adrenaline, cortisol and a sensitised nervous system.

Picking up this book is such a brave thing to do, especially as this 'fight-or-flight' response wants all of your attention. It makes you feel like something awful is about to happen, usually to do with our minds, our bodies, or related to something we have been worrying about recently. The anxious response likes to throw some uncomfortable physical symptoms your way, such as nausea, a fast heart rate, muscle tension (all over the body), just to name a few. It also likes to crank up the speed of our thoughts, as well as provide us with a flood of emotions, such as fear, terror, sadness and anger. Sounds fun right?

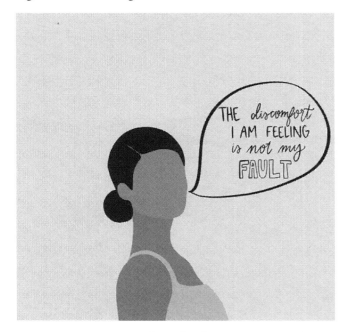

@simplysophiedesigns

We know how difficult it can be to explore the scary topic of anxiety. However, rest assured that this book has been carefully curated to be a reassuring manual for anxious sufferers. We have created this as a warm, hope-inspiring resource for people who suffer from anxiety and anxiety-related disorders. These are the people who are exhausted by worry, perhaps about external matters, or worrying about their own sanity, or *why* they are even worrying – a fear of their own fear.

You have probably picked up this book because you have been experiencing many uncomfortable symptoms of anxiety. Some of the most common and scary symptoms we work with (and have experienced ourselves) are living with an unwanted sense of fear and a constant feeling that something bad is about to happen – a sense of continuous dread. Perhaps you're feeling a bit detached from yourself and the world, or even from yourself and your body? This is a phenomenon called Derealisation. It's likely that you have a heightened awareness of your senses, where everything seems brighter around you. You may zone in on the slightest sounds around you and start to feel detached from the situation that you are in, almost like you are not there and you are observing the situation.

Catastrophic thoughts such as 'what if' statements: 'What if I can't breathe?' or 'what if I am having a heart attack?' start to pop up and stick in your mind, increasing the anxiety levels with every irrational thought. There's a good chance you have spiralling negative thoughts that seem to 'stick in your mind', where no matter how much you try not to think of them, they just seem to stick around. Not being able to rid the thought increases your anxiety, right? Trust us when we say this: we have been there too.

Maybe you are prone to bouts of panic, where we become scared that we are about to lose our ability to breath, feel like we are about to collapse, have a heart attack, or lose our minds? Furthermore, you may experience an increased heart rate and shallow breathing, sometimes out of nowhere, making you feel on edge, where the more you think of it, the more you can feel your heart racing, causing you to perspire and your palms to become sweaty. This is very common and is central to what are commonly known as bouts of panic, or 'panic attacks', although we don't like to use the term 'attack' because the term is biologically inaccurate.

If you feel anxious or panicky right now, just know that nothing is attacking you. You are safe. It just *feels* dangerous. We assure you that this feeling will pass.

Anxiety is such a broad condition and it involves many strange and uncomfortable symptoms. We have split anxiety into separate sections and common diagnoses to help you to conceptualise *your* anxious presentation. As a psychotherapist, Josh often works with various presentations of anxiety. A proportion of the clients he sees actually come with diagnoses from doctors or psychiatrists. Whilst he feels there is too much medicalisation of the mental health field, he does believe in the value of disordered anxiety having certain terms to help us to identify common presentations of excessive anxiety. Here are some examples of common anxiety-related conditions:

Just to be clear, we are not diagnosing you, we are just using these terms to show you many common presentations of anxiety. We invite you to make a note, in your mind or on paper, of which of these apply to you:

Panic Disorder, or Fear of Panic

Panic disorder occurs when we become frightened of anxiety and panic attacks. Furthermore, we may not know why we are panicking, so we may spend a lot of time trying to work out what is 'wrong' with us. People who fear panic will almost always avoid doing things for fear that they may go insane, or that something awful might happen. The most common excuse for avoiding that we hear is "I avoid just in case I have a panic attack."

Do you get those thoughts of 'what if I'm on my own and I suddenly get anxious, what will I do?' or 'what if I'm out with friends, or out in a restaurant, or driving, or sat at my work desk and anxiety suddenly kicks in? What if I start to go crazy and everyone around me sees this horrible feeling - that I battle with constantly - come flooding out of me?' Or, one of the main ones we hear, "what if I can't cope?"

Most people who have this type of anxiety tend to experience their first wave of panic from seemingly out of nowhere. This frightens them so much that they withdraw and commit all of their time to trying to prevent another wave of panic from happening again; thereby causing a negative thought cycle that keeps anxiety and panic at the centre of their lives. We'll talk more about panic later in the book. If this applies to you, fear not, as anxiety can be overcome!

5

Health Anxiety

This is when we end up in an anxious terrifying cycle where we often *misinterpret* symptoms of anxiety as symptoms of something catastrophic. Do you find yourself googling every little symptom and coming to the worst-case scenario? That little twitch you noticed on your arm a few times suddenly becomes a possibly life altering condition? Where all at the click of a button this one irrational thought becomes an obsession and every time you google to research further you get 'more evidence' that something is seriously wrong? We wrote this book at the time of a pandemic and can't tell you the amount of times we interpreted a simple cough, or a sneeze, as a virus that could kill us.

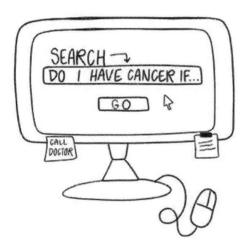

@simplysophiedesigns

Social Anxiety

Do you ever find your mind going blank when you are mid-sentence and then find yourself getting anxious because you can't remember what you were talking about? When you are out in crowds of people, does it ever feel like everyone is staring at you and almost like time has slowed down? If you are familiar with one of Dean's favourite films, 'The Truman Show', it's similar to that moment where Truman starts to think everyone is watching his every move.

Many people with social anxiety will spend hours anticipating attending an event, or even spend hours replaying conversations in their minds after the event has happened. They are prone to misinterpreting others' facial expressions, or worried that they have offended someone, or fear being perceived as uninteresting. Obviously, this is anxiety and a nasty trick; you have value. You have worth!

Agoraphobia

People with agoraphobia tend to stick to their 'safe spaces' because they fear how they will feel outside of them, or believe that something awful might happen if they venture 'too far'. The most common safe spaces are our homes (even just our bedrooms), the areas around our homes, a relative or loved one's house, or our workplace. People who get anxious on the road (driving anxiety) can often convince themselves that certain routes are 'safe' so they stick to those. Many people have often had their first wave of panic in the car, which has often resulted in agoraphobia. Agoraphobia, in a nutshell, is the fear of being overwhelmed outside of a perceived 'safe space'.

Intrusive Thoughts

Have you ever had horrendous, unwanted thoughts that trigger and provoke anxiety? The content of intrusive thoughts knows no boundaries, where horrible images – usually of a taboo nature – creep their way into our minds and we categorically do not want them there. The most common intrusive thoughts include thoughts of a sexual or violent nature, usually to do with loved ones, or harm to self. Intrusive thoughts are very normal; everybody experiences them. However, for anxious people, they can become sticky and lead us into questioning their nature, or origins, which in turn leads us into questioning our own sanity or mental state.

Obsessive Compulsive Disorder (OCD)

Do you live out physical or mental rituals in order to prevent an imagined disaster from happening? Are you obsessed with cleanliness just in case you may contaminate someone? OCD thrives off the belief that "if we don't do X, then the awful catastrophe Y, will happen…" Some common examples are obsessive cleaning, checking plugs, skin picking, hair pulling, enacting a strict routine at certain times of the day, or even completing an entirely 'mental' routine played out in our minds. No matter what the content associated with OCD, it is very treatable and manageable. That said, working directly with an OCD specialist and having an OCD specific book will perhaps be of added benefit.

Generalised Anxiety Disorder (GAD)

We are no strangers to GAD. Generalised Anxiety presents as a constant worry with a multitude of topics to worry about. We may even be worrying about the state of worrying itself! People with GAD live out most days with a constant sense of unease, focussing intensely on their thoughts (what if?s), their feelings and the strange sensations that come with anxiety.

Post-Traumatic Stress

Anxiety can surface in people as a result of unprocessed trauma. If this is the case, then we believe that professional help and guidance is mandatory, as this book alone will not be sufficient, nor can it offer a grounding presence should difficult memories arise as a result of the trauma. That said, PTSD can be treated and it is also really helpful to learn about PTSD to demystify its presentation and symptoms.

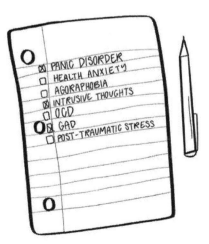

@simplysophiedesigns

...What now?

Anxiety has many other presentations, but these we found to be the most common. We are confident the principles we outline in this book will help you, regardless of how your anxiety manifests. If you can relate to any of these, then we believe that this book will be able to help you. If you have answered yes to many of these statements, or somehow nodded your head in agreement, then this book is for you. If you have answered yes to only a few of these statements, then this is book for you too, or even if you can resonate with only one. If you haven't answered yes to any of the above, then our guess is that you have picked this book up to better understand a loved one, a friend, family member or co-worker, so I will say it again, this book is for you too: in such cases this book can definitely be helpful.

Meet the Authors

We are Joshua Fletcher, psychotherapist, and Dean Stott of DLC Anxiety and we can confidently state that we are well versed in both working with anxiety and experiencing it ourselves! We are two young(ish) men from Manchester, UK, who have both suffered from anxiety disorders in the past and worked through them to get to the positions we are in now. Joshua Fletcher (@anxietyjosh on Instagram) is a qualified psychotherapist specialising in working with anxiety and anxiety-related conditions and runs his private practice called *The Panic Room* in Manchester. Joshua is also a best-selling author of previous self-help books, *Anxiety: Panicking about Panic (Createspace)* and *Anxiety: Practical about Panic (John Murray Press)*. He is also co-host of the popular anxiety podcast, *The Panic Pod*.

Dean Stott of *DLC Anxiety* runs the largest anxiety support community on Instagram (@DLCanxiety) which, at the time of writing, has amassed over 900,000 followers from all around the globe. Dean has studied Psychology at University and holds diplomas in Life Coaching and Cognitive Behavioural Therapy for Anxiety, Depression and Phobias. Further to Dean's academic background, he has also overcome panic disorder and believes that this personal experience of overcoming anxiety really resonates with his Instagram community. By promoting an open dialogue on his platform, he believes that people dealing with an anxiety disorder can feel less alone; they can listen to what works for other people and also share what works for them. DLC Anxiety is a worldwide virtual community centre, where everyone comes together to support each other on their own journey to recovery. Dean also enjoys interviewing people about mental health, including relevant professionals and celebrities.

We are privileged to be to be able to share our knowledge and expertise to as many people who will listen. Yes, we have the professional and academic backgrounds, but we have walked in similar shoes and share a lot in common with you. We are just further down the recovery path at the moment and we have written this book to help guide the way. The book has been created to share the knowledge we have gained that has helped us, and we are sharing it with you because we understand just how scary it can be when you feel trapped in your own mind. Ultimately, we understand how terrifying it can be when your mind runs faster than you. We understand how difficult it can be when your mind has become entangled within itself and everything feels confusing. Let us try and help you to untangle that anxiety.

We know what it's like when you wake up and start to wonder when the anxiety will start to kick in, then when it does kick in, it feels like the battle for the day has commenced. Have you ever woken up not feeling anxious, then infuriatingly, made yourself anxious because it felt strange not to be anxious in that moment? Well, we have been there too!

How about if we told you it may feel like a battle but it's not? How would those words sit with you? This is by no means us belittling the anxiety you are feeling. This is us shining a big light on the anxiety and saying "Hey we know your tricks, and we are about to pass on that knowledge to our readers, so you better be ready, because when they face you next time, they will start to see the cracks."

Dean

When Dean was in the middle of panic disorder, he turned to a very dear friend of his for reassurance. They had spoken a little in the past about anxiety and he was aware that he used to struggle with anxiety in his 20's and early 30's. Dean's friend is now 42 and living anxiety disorder free. His words carried weight. When Dean was telling him how he was feeling and what symptoms he was experiencing, his friend would reply with examples from his past when he used to feel exactly the same. Dean's friend would help him feel like he was speaking from his perspective – like he had walked in his shoes. This experience felt more valuable than any doctor's appointment. That said, the doctor had been an excellent place to start, in ensuring his symptoms were anxiety related by ruling out other conditions that could cause similar symptoms, but once these had been ruled out, he had felt like his options were limited.

Dean was offered medication, told the benefits of exercise, healthy eating, mindfulness and self-help CBT and was sent on his way to figure out his own journey to recovery. Yes, each one of these options were proven to reduce anxiety levels but he needed more. Ultimately, Dean needed a way out of the constant overthinking, the constant worrying about when might the next panic attack occur. He didn't want to wake up in the morning and have the first thing on his mind be anxiety. He wanted to feel how his friend did; there was a desire to feel like 'pre-anxious Dean' and he worried if this was even possible anymore?

The knowledge Dean gained from his friend was the number one reason that he was able to help himself break free from an ongoing cycle of panic and worrying about thoughts and sensations.

"I am forever grateful to my friend for telling me that anxiety wasn't going to send me crazy and that I wasn't always going to feel this way. Even though I felt stuck in an anxious spiral of irrational thoughts and fear, I was grateful that there was a light at the end of the tunnel. That everything was going to be okay. I will always remember my friend's words 'If I came out of it, you can too." That really stuck with me. My friend was no different to me, we were both in the same job living similar lives yet he was able to wake up and the first thing on his mind would be food and not anxiety. I must admit the second thought on my mind was food!" - Dean

Dean wants to bottle this feeling of hope that he received and pass it on to as many people who would listen. He also wants to share with you the tips that would help him reduce anxiety or not focus on irrational thoughts. Like Dean, you can trial and error each technique and use the one best for you.

"His words were priceless; he truly did pick me up and guide me on my journey to recovery." - Dean

Dean now spreads his positive words of hope through interviewing experts in the industry on his large social media platform, as well as hosting his own podcast.

Josh

After recovering from panic disorder and agoraphobia in 2013, Joshua decided to write down his experience of overcoming anxiety in his first self-published book, Anxiety: Panicking about Panic. With no expectations about its release, Josh continued his then career of working with children with emotional and behavioural difficulties. On checking his emails a few weeks later, Josh was awe-struck at how many copies of his book had sold within the first few weeks. The news soon started to spread and even to this day *Panicking about Panic* still tops the Amazon best-selling charts as a self-published book.

"I recall being at work one day then suddenly it felt like my whole reality had changed. I had this weird feeling of detachment, a huge sense of dread and I froze. I was terrified about what was happening to me and thought I'd lost my mind. I went home and became scared to leave the house for weeks. I constantly tried to 'work out my feelings' and just tried to wait for the feelings to disappear. Obviously this didn't work. I had never felt so alone!" - Josh

This inspired Josh to a career change and he began studying anxiety and the psychology around it in more depth. He trained to become a Psychotherapist, completing his MSc in Counselling Psychology and a PGCert in Cognitive Behavioural Therapy. To this day, he has worked with hundreds of people to successfully overcome a multitude of anxiety-related conditions. His second book, *Anxiety: Practical about Panic*, was published by Hachette and his reputation as the go-to person for Anxiety grows by the day. Josh has worked with the BBC, Worldwide FM, MIND and many well-known consumer brands.

Josh took to Instagram under the name 'AnxietyJosh' and met fellow ex-sufferer Dean of DLCanxiety where they quickly bonded over a lot of shared experiences. After some engaging interviews and many positives talks, they decided to co-write a book. There was the added serendipity that two men, of similar age, from the same city, have met at a point in their lives where they are both ready to convey a message to help others.

"This is a lovely opportunity to work with someone who actually 'gets it' and we're so excited to share what we know with the world." – Josh

In Conversation

Josh: What can you tell us about your experience with anxiety Dean?

Dean: So, myself I had general anxiety disorder, like a mixture of general anxiety disorder and panic disorder, oh and a mix of health anxiety in there. So, how it started was um after the passing of my father and, like any male does, I kept the emotions in and tried to just get on with life, almost put it to the back of my mind.

Josh: How did keeping emotions in work for you? [Laughter].

Dean: Yeah, well what happened was yeah, two three months down the line I remember just being in the middle of the shopping center because it's one thing that I enjoy doing - going shopping. Low and behold out of nowhere was just this huge sense of impending doom like something was seriously wrong with me like...

Josh: Oh yeah, I could relate to that. Yeah, was it like when your vision just goes a bit weird and you're like, "Whoa I don't feel here."?

Dean: It was like that and it was like, do you know you've mentioned it before in the past- you know that *whoosh* feeling? So, you can just be doing what you normally do and then it's just a completely different feeling that almost takes over your body.

Josh: Oh, the *whoosh.*

Dean: Yes.

Josh: Yeah, like it's the perfect description like a woosh- [**Dean:** Yes] what's happened here, but in response to nothing, because we know the shopping center for you is not dangerous.

Chapter 2

What is Anxiety?

Featured Illustrator: @katies.self.care.diaries

Let's strip it right to the bone and ask the question: *what is anxiety?*

Anxiety is a *feeling* of unease that includes emotions such as worry or fear. Anxiety can be measured on a spectrum that can be anything from feeling slightly nervous to struggling with acute panic. Every human on the planet has feelings of anxiety at some point in their life and there are lots of common examples of *conventional* anxiety, such as:

- Worrying about sitting an exam

- Worrying about test results

- Worrying about that upcoming job interview

- Nervous about a first date

- General worries about your relationship

- Worrying and ruminating about the future

During times like these, feeling anxious can feel completely normal. Nerves are known to help us focus and perform better, or to help us problem-solve. Try and consider how you felt before an interview, or a driving test. We can all feel the effects of anxiety, but we don't really worry about *why* we are anxious – we are just anxious because we care about the outcome. It is ok to feel anxious in anticipation of something that we care about and it can actually be performance-enhancing for many of us.

Anxiety is an intense and induced response to things that may make us fearful. Normally the brain monitors our fear and anxiety without allowing it to interrupt our daily lives. Our brains are automatically scanning the area around us and, if there is a nearby threat, our brains will respond by increasing our anxiety and fear accordingly.

For some people this area of the brain functions more than it should do; this being a form of excessive anxiety that can be overwhelming and that interferes with daily life. The person will experience many symptoms and may start to develop many irrational behaviours.

Anxiety that persists and lasts for a long time like this may be classified as an *anxiety disorder.*

When does Anxiety become a problem then?

Anxiety becomes problematic when it becomes *excessive* or, in psychology terms, "disordered". Anxiety can creep into our lives and cause huge disorder – disrupting our normal lives, behaviours and routines. Feelings of anxiety can become very acute and suddenly we can become concerned about an array of symptoms associated with how we feel. Disordered anxiety occurs when we stop worrying about issues in the external world and focus all of our attention on our 'internal world'; this world within us consisting of three parts:

1. Feelings

With excessive anxiety, we can often experience feelings of doom, or dread, that feel like a heavy cloud over our existence. We can feel very 'on-edge', scared and, on occasions, terrified. We may feel like we are not in our own bodies, as if we are observing ourselves exist in an alternative reality. Alongside feelings of fear, we may also feel down, helpless and notice a lingering sadness. Furthermore, we may also experience feelings of frustration, anger and irritability.

2. Thoughts

Anxiety comes with a boat load of thoughts that can often rush into our minds faster than we can comprehend them. What's interesting though, is that you can distinguish between a 'normal' thought and an 'anxious' thought by how each thought begins: almost every anxious thought begins with a "what if...?", followed by scary and catastrophic content derived from our imaginations. Anxious thoughts follow this simple formula:

What if {insert catastrophe} happens?

Some of the most common 'what if...?'s we hear are:

- What if I have another panic attack?

- What if I never feel normal again?

- What if I am broken?

- What if I am freaking out, or going crazy?

- What if they are judging me?

- What if I have a heart attack?

- What if I can't sustain this feeling and it eventually hurts me?

'What if…?'s are just thoughts. However, when you combine them with feelings and sensations, they suddenly seem more real – anxiety's best and only trick!

3. Sensations

On top of feelings and thoughts, anxiety comes with a multitude of physical symptoms and sensations. There are so, so many! Some of the most common sensations associated with anxiety are: feelings of detachment from reality (derealisation), a pounding heart, tight chest, headaches or a 'tight band' feeling around the head, nausea, symptoms similar to irritable bowel syndrome, sweating, shaking, a sensitivity to light, muscle tension all over the body, chest 'flutters' or the heart 'skipping a beat', torso pains, muscle twitching, jaw tension and bloating – just to name a few!

We are no strangers to these symptoms ourselves and have suffered with many of the examples from all three parts of anxiety. We recommend taking time to write down the different facets of your anxiety, just to help you conceptualise what is happening with you.

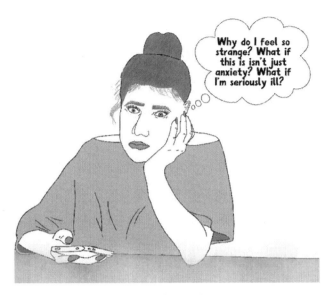

@katies.self.care.diaries

How Common is Anxiety?

Anxiety is very common, despite most people struggling with it feeling isolated and somehow 'different' to people around them. Anxiety Disorders affect around 18% of the population in the US every year, which means around 1 in 5 people will, at some point, struggle with anxiety in some way, namely a combination of the *Thoughts, Feelings* and *Sensations* mentioned before. If there are 20 of you in a room, then 4 of you will experience disordered anxiety at some point in your life. In the UK, where we are from, 6.6% of people will be experiencing some form of disordered anxiety in a given week.

There is no definitive answer as to why anxiety has increased over the years. Many researchers believe it is a combination of many factors that have contributed to the increase, including: the impact of social media on self-esteem and how we value ourselves, poor sleeping habits, lowered stigma and under reporting in the past. Perhaps it has always been there, but we were all just suffering in silence?

The DLC Anxiety platform was born on Instagram. Dean is so happy to have been able to create a worldwide platform that's shining the brightest light on anxiety and panic disorder, and using social media for its purpose: to spread awareness and connect people together under one umbrella, trying to ensure nobody ever feels that they are alone. Fortunately, the platform has enabled many people to come together and share their experiences. It surprised us… the sheer amount of people that can relate to feeling anxious.

It is amazing to see such influential people on social media using their platforms to create mental health awareness. Popstars such as Madison Beer, who has a huge following, regularly posts psychoeducational posts and speaks out about her own mental health and urges her fans to speak out and seek help for their own. Along with being an actor, comedian and podcast host, the super talented Brittany Furlan Lee regularly urges people to speak about their own mental health and, if they are struggling, to seek help. Brittany also gives her followers an insight into her own life, often telling followers when she is feeling anxious or has just had a panic attack. We also loved the interview with Alessia Cara that we hosted on the platform, as well as the ones with Jude Moore, Lily Cornell Silver and many others. The interviews demonstrated that anxiety can affect us all from all walks of life.

Anxiety vs Anxiety Disorder

Anxiety is a term that gets bandied around a lot, much to the displeasure of people who are crippled by it. It can often be referred to as an exaggerated term for something that was only mildly anxiety provoking. For example, a person playfully startles a friend and the friend responds with "oh my god you gave me a panic attack!". Furthermore, diagnostic labels are loosely given to normal character traits, such as labelling someone who likes to be organised as "wow he is so OCD!". People who experience actual panic attacks, or suffer with Obsessive Compulsive Disorder, will tell you that it is nothing to joke about. We found when discussing the writing of this book that it is incredibly important to distinguish between everyday anxiety and *disordered* anxiety.

Anxiety and anxiety disorders often get confused and it is this confusion that can continue to fuel the false narrative that anxiety is just something we all deal with and that those who openly speak about anxiety are somehow weak or attention seeking. This couldn't be further from the truth, because having an anxiety disorder and facing anxiety each day takes strength and courage.

It is important to note that anxiety, as an emotion and a biological response, is a healthy phenomenon that we all experience (we'll discuss this more in depth later). However, when anxiety becomes excessive, overwhelming, chronic and debilitating, it can start to affect our day to day life. This is when anxiety creeps into *disorder* territory. An anxiety disorder happens when anxiety becomes overwhelming or appears unexpectedly. Anxiety disorders are a mental condition and can have a huge impact on your day to day life.

To reiterate, anxiety is *a natural response* that we all have from time to time and, in the right situation, anxiety can be useful. For example, just before an exam a person may get anxious, however this type of anxiety can help keep you focused. A sports person feels the adrenaline before a big match; a spokesperson riles themselves up for a convincing pitch; nerves during a musical performance help us to unlock a higher level of performance. However, someone who is diagnosed with an anxiety *disorder* may ruminate over the exam weeks before; it may consume their minds on a daily basis causing physical and emotional symptoms. Right before and during the exam they will experience intense symptoms of anxiety.

"Anxiety is fleeting whereas an anxiety disorder is constant and can occur over a period of weeks, months or even years." - Dean

A doctor or psychologist can diagnose an anxiety disorder, or many people just seem to self-diagnose. Either way, it is always helpful to acknowledge an anxiety problem and we have written this book to help you as much as we can.

Common Pitfalls of Anxiety

1 Trying to 'Fix' Anxiety

One of the biggest mistakes people make is assuming they are *broken*, or that something is wrong with them. The anxious response is a healthy, normal response, however, when it becomes excessive, or disordered, many people jump to the conclusion that something has 'broken' them in some way, or that they need fixing. The person who is dealing with anxiety will often try and find solutions 'to fix the situation'. As humans, we have a tendency to want to fix something if we are unable to manage it successfully.

The problem with trying to fix anxiety is that you are not broken in the first place. Highlighting that there's a problem that needs to be fixed, is the equivalent to shining a big, bright spotlight on the anxiety we may be feeling. In turn, this means we are giving the anxiety more attention and fuelling the constant loop of anxious thoughts and behaviours. Anxiety occurs in response to a perceived or actual threat: our minds can't process the difference between perceived or real and will react in the exact same way.

People who fall into this category will often have shelves full of self-help books, saved documents of reassurance from social media and non-fiction outlets and will often avoid doing things until "I feel better".

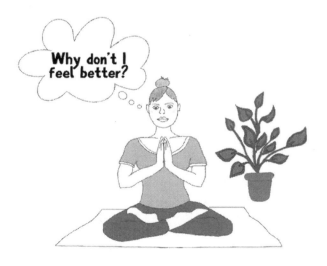

@katies.self.care.diaries

2. Avoidance

Avoidance is one of the main reasons why we can remain in an anxious cycle. As soon as we start avoiding things, the brain notices that we start *behaving* unusually and gets *tricked* into thinking something is wrong. People with anxiety begin to avoid places, or people, for fear of triggering their anxious response, or believing that they will pass out, or have a heart attack, or go crazy, etc.

"I honestly spent a month in my bedroom waiting for the feelings to pass. What I didn't realise is that this was not helping. Once I realised that avoiding doing things was only contributing to the anxiety, and that anxiety itself wasn't dangerous, I started to reintroduce my old life back." - Josh

An example of this would be: if someone has a panic disorder and their trigger is a shopping mall, then every time they go and do their grocery shopping, they get intense anxiety which often leads to panic attacks. Then they may start to change their behaviour to try and reduce the anxiety they are feeling. This may start with going to the mall at quieter times or limiting the time they are in the shop. Initially, they may find some short-term relief from intense anxiety, but what this behaviour is doing is conditioning the mind to think that every time they go to the shopping mall, they may be in danger.

What you tend to find is that the anxiety will start to get more intense, this can then lead to further behaviour such as changing shopping habits altogether and shopping online. Again, this may give some *temporary* relief to the person, but this learnt behaviour is *conditioning* the mind to think that shopping malls are now a threat. This can then progress to the mind thinking that every time the person leaves their home, they are under threat, so anxiety may start to pop up when the person is outside. This can have a huge impact on someone's life and can lead to Agoraphobia, which is a fear of being in situations where escape may be difficult, or help may not be available if something was to go wrong.

3 Google Searching

Another common pitfall that we hear often and can relate to is the dreaded *google search*: googling symptoms and believing the ever so insightful 'Dr Google'. In a world dominated by technology, it's just too easy to reach for your phone and type in whatever symptom may have been bothering you that day. The only problem is that google is not programmed to give you the most likely medical cause for the symptom you have searched, it is programmed to give you the most searched or talked about conditions, so you will see conditions such as cancer, heart problems, neurological disorders, tumours etc.

What does this do for an anxious mind? Cue the rabbit hole: an anxious mind will zone in on the worst-case scenario, dismissing all other likely causes and look for further 'evidence' that what they have is a life-threatening illness. This can consume someone's daily life with constant worry and 'what if' thoughts. This common pitfall is also a symptom of health anxiety.

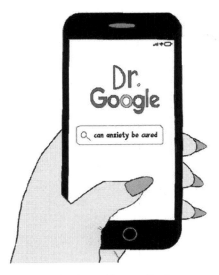

@katies.self.care.diaries

4 The Miracle Thought / Trying to work out anxiety

A big pitfall that people fall into is trying to intellectualise the problem, by trying to 'work out' their anxiety by exploring their thoughts and ruminating on the possibility that we can 'work out' how we feel by thinking our way out of it. In Josh's practice, he calls this *Inception* thinking – a reference to the Hollywood film that has multiple dream levels in a convoluted plot that has baffled a lot of people. In reality, we aren't searching the deeper levels of our minds for an answer though, we are simply contributing to an anxious cycle and subscribing to a false belief that we are broken in some way.

5 Reliance on others

Do you ever feel scared to be left on your own? Scared that you might get anxious and not have anyone there with you to rely on? If your answer to this question is 'yes' then you are not alone! Reliance, or co-dependency, is a common pitfall that we see with anxious people. Reliance to have someone there 'just in case you get anxious' or the fear of 'being left alone and you might go crazy' are statements that we have heard a lot and thoughts we have had over the years. What you will find as you continue to read, is that anxiety may have different disguises, but it always has the same results when it appears. If we show it too much attention, it will peak, but then it always goes away.

Rest assured, we are never in a constant state of fixed anxiety: it's not biologically possible!

If we become reliant on people, then when we are alone, we start to become more anxious. What we are doing is training the brain to think that when we are alone, we must be in some sense of danger. With this perceived threat our body will do what it is supposed to do and increase our anxiety levels. Unfortunately, this can develop even further into avoidance and an anxious cycle; we only have to imagine being left alone and we may feel our anxiety starting to rise.

6 We asked others

We asked the *DLC Platform* what common pitfalls they have experienced when trying to manage anxiety and here is what they said. Can you relate to any of these?

"Substance abuse, I used to drink heavily when I was feeling anxious, it sort of helped at the time because it numbed my mind, but what I found was that when I woke up the next day, I would have the worst anxiety and this would be an ongoing cycle of increased anxiety."

"Pushing myself to do something I didn't want to do, all just in case it reduces anxiety which it never does. I now know this is called 'white-knuckling'."

"Trying to become anxiety free, you hear so many books and people state that you can live anxiety free."

"I have been worried about the virus and falling victim to being consumed by the news, which I know is only fuelling anxiety further."

"I used to always get thoughts that would pop into my head and stick there, I always tried to not think something, when I did this it just made the anxiety worse."

"Deep breathing and concentrating on my breath, when I have a panic attack the first thing that changes is my breathing. I used to always try to overcome this and do all the textbook breathing exercises only to find out it would make the anxiety worse."

Some examples that Josh has heard from his readers and clients from *The Panic Room* (with permission) are:

"I've tried yoga and meditation for my anxiety and it didn't help."

"I've cut out all unhealthy foods and even cut out gluten in the hope that it would make me feel better."

"I've tried the holistic approach to anxiety. I've sampled every essential oil, herbal remedy, special tea and even tried reiki and gong baths to try and help my anxiety."

"I exercise twice a day but it still doesn't shift how I feel."

Interestingly, all these approaches subscribe to the narrative that we need to 'fix' or 'do something' when we are anxious. In the following chapter, we will explain why we do this, as well as the important question of *why* we get anxious and what anxiety actually is.

In Conversation

Josh: I had it in work, which was a place I was very comfortable in, then suddenly *whoosh*! Oh my god! I started to become really scared after mine though. What about you?

Dean: I did. So, I was in the center of the shopping center and all the what-if thoughts were just telling me, "What if I am in immediate danger?" You need to get out of the shopping center. So, I almost ran out of the shopping center and back to my car, knowing that that was like a safe place for me, if you know what I mean?"

Josh: So, you weren't worrying about your dodgy dress sense?

Dean: I wasn't no, not on this occasion [laughter]. But yeah, as anxiety does, it reached a peak and then by the time I got to my car, I felt that the anxiety started to decrease. But that was my first real panic attack and that's what really kick-started the panic disorder.

Josh: It's interesting because for me it is always the word *misinterpretation* that applies. I misinterpreted my initial anxiety. I spent months at home trying to work out my anxiety, and I was just keeping this anxious threat response on all the time, getting scary what-ifs, scary sensations. And just kind of regressing into a bit of a depression as well, because it was affecting my life. Yeah, scary when - I don't know about you - but I just didn't know who to turn to at the time. No one got it. It's really strange trying to say to someone, "Yeah, I don't kind of feel like I'm here. I feel petrified for no reason and having weird thoughts and sensations, because they just look at you like, 'What?"

Dean: Exactly. And that's a really good point saying that, really when you first experience it and from myself and speaking to other people who've gone through anxiety disorders- when you first experience it you really don't know who to turn to.

And I remember, I was even scared of going to the doctors because I had in my mind that this must be something serious, this must be something that's seriously wrong with me. And the anxiety was a feeling that I didn't want to find out more about.

Chapter 3

Why do we get the Anxious Response?

Featured illustrator: @selfcarevisuals

The Amygdala

Have you ever stepped into the road and noticed, at the last second, a car was driving straight towards you, so you instantly jolted back to the curb? Perhaps your heart felt like it was in your stomach, your breathing intensified and you could feel your heart racing? This is the anxious response. It was anxiety that saved you from getting hit by that car.

Anxiety is crucial for our survival. It is our body's natural response - a fear system built within us to keep us safe. Without it, we wouldn't have evolved to where we are now. Our ancestors would have been attacked and killed in the wild if we didn't have this inbuilt protection system. We needed to be constantly on alert, hypervigilant and in a state of anticipation to apprehend potential predators, such as lions, sabre-tooth tigers, snakes and people trying to sell you life insurance.

It is paramount that we understand the role of the anxious response when it comes to eradicating *excessive* anxiety.

"When learning about anxiety and overcoming it, we always start with the oldest part of our brain: our lizard brain. Within the lizard brain, there is a part called the amygdala. It is this part, the amygdala, where we always, always begin." - Josh

Have you ever experienced the sensation of falling when you're about to drift off to sleep? Where you're in a kind of half asleep, half-awake state and you visualise and feel like you're tripping over, or falling off a pavement? If you have, you'll know that you jolt yourself awake immediately and feel a bit shocked. Much like the car in the road analogy, this is the amygdala at work.

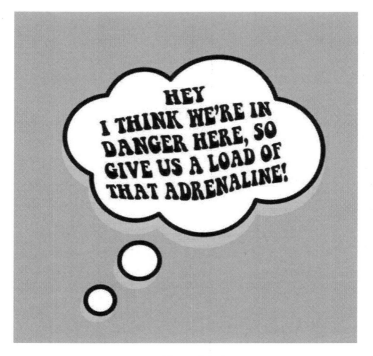

@selfcarevisuals

The amygdala is the oldest and fastest part of our brains, but it isn't the smartest. Its primary job is to look out for danger by constantly scanning things using our senses. We all have an amygdala, it is inbuilt and is absolutely vital for survival. If you have had a friend or family member who has frightened you as a joke – saying "boo!" for example - then you'll notice you'll feel shocked, then on-edge, and it takes a few moments to calm down. The amygdala reacted before you could, engaging a defensive response just in case there was danger. Once you and the amygdala determined that there was no danger, you calmed down again.

The same applies when watching a scary moment in a horror film, or if you suddenly have to slam on the brakes in a car. This is the common function of the amygdala. It turns on and off in response to perceived 'danger' and it does it very quickly. Ultimately, the amygdala is the *conductor* of the fear response. It is the "on switch", the boss, the CEO of *Fear Inc.* and it can be annoying as hell when things become disordered. After all, most people reading this book will often be experiencing an anxious response that triggers in response to little or no danger.

It is really important to understand what happens when the amygdala decides there is danger and what it does to change our bodies in response to said danger. It is this process that helps many people understand and motivate themselves to overcome excessive and disordered anxiety. Remember, the amygdala triggers the fear response when it *perceives* danger; whether or not there is *actual* danger does not matter. If the amygdala perceives there is danger, then it will activate!

If the amygdala decides there is danger, it communicates very quickly with a part of our brain called *hypothalamus*. It is this part of our brain that triggers *the sympathetic nervous system*, which is responsible for releasing *adrenaline* and making us feel fear, 'on-edge' and panic. The amygdala says to the hypothalamus "hey I think we're in danger here, so give us a load of that adrenaline!" Anxious people can notice this when they feel a 'whoosh' feeling, or that feeling like there's a pit in our stomach, or "butterflies' as many people describe it. This is basically anxiety!

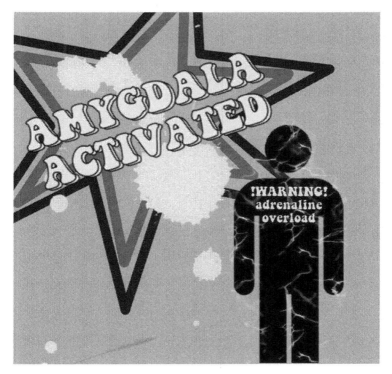

@selfcarevisuals

But why do we experience it when we don't want to? Why do we experience it in the absence of any perceivable danger? Let's look at the anxious response a bit more:

We experience the world through our thoughts and senses. All sensory information, from our vision, sounds, taste and touch, is sent to the 'motherboard' of our brains: the *thalamus*. This is like the main operations centre of our brains and this is where anxiety starts:

"I like to think of the thalamus as the main call centre, or telephone switchboard of the brain, where messages and calls are directed and redirected to the appropriate places of the brain. A bit like "Operator, which service do you require?" - Josh

The thalamus then sends this sensory information onto the *neo-cortex*, which is our 'thinking brain'. It is when information is sent to our thinking brain that we decide whether or not this sensory stimulus is 'dangerous' or not. From here, a message is sent to the amygdala, which then produces an 'appropriate' emotional response, such as fear, terror, upset or anger. If our thinking brain deems the situation dangerous, then it tells the amygdala to signal the hypothalamus to release adrenaline and trigger the sympathetic nervous system.

For example, you're walking down a street when you see a dog coming towards you. From far away the dog looks harmless, but it still has your attention. Our visual sense is telling the thalamus what it is seeing and, because we like dogs, we become excited or happy to see the dog. To us, this is the appropriate response to have because we like dogs (in this example anyway).

However, as we get closer, we notice that the dog is showing its teeth, and is foaming at the mouth. Its eyes are red and we realise it is walking erratically. We also notice that it is growling. This dog could be potentially rabid and dangerous. Our visual and auditory senses now take this new information and present it to the thalamus, which then relays the information to the amygdala. The amygdala would now deem that this dog is no longer something to be happy about, but something to be *afraid* of! The amygdala then signals to the hypothalamus to release adrenaline. We then experience fear and are flooded with catastrophic thoughts about the dog biting us, which in turn makes us avoid the dog – perhaps by crossing over the road or turning around and walking away. This is the *fight-or-flight* response at work.

However, and this bit is important, if we are faced with an imminent danger, then the thalamus will send sensory information *directly* to the amygdala, just in case we need to fight, run or freeze. This occurred when you tried to cross the road, but there was a car speeding towards you. This quickfire message from the thalamus, directly to the amygdala, occurred when your friend startled you, or you had a 'falling dream' as you tried to drift off to sleep. Using our dog analogy, this occurs when the dog suddenly jumps out the bushes and dives towards you catching you unaware. The signal from the thalamus directly to the amygdala is a *rapid* response and it has to be. It is this response that saved your life and can save your life again. However, it can be an annoyance and uncomfortable when it triggers unnecessarily.

Scientists, until only recently, used to believe that the 'amygdala' alone was the central part that served fear and anxiety. Previous studies had shown that monkeys with a damaged amygdala were fearless in the face of danger. In people with an anxiety disorder, scientists were under the assumption that increased and disruptive anxiety and fear were caused by a hyperactive amygdala.

However, today scientists know that it is not solely the amygdala that is at play and that it is a fear *network*; a constant chatter between different regions within the brain. By splitting the brain into two sections: a *cognitive brain* and an *emotional brain*, we can better understand this. The frontal part of the brain where our thoughts are processed and our sensations experienced is the cognitive brain. The amygdala is located deep inside the brain and is part of the *emotional* brain. It is believed we only fear anxiety when signals from the emotional brain overpower the cognitive brain and flow into our consciousness. To use an example, imagine that you were anxious and floating in deep sea water. We know that attacks by sea creatures whilst in the sea are rare, but for some people, treading water and feeling anxious can trigger a multitude of fears (the emotional brain). However, let's say we're treading water next to a boat for safety, then the cognitive brain network can overtake the emotional network and dampen the fear response.

In summary, the anxious response can override current thinking and logic; it can bypass asking the neo-cortex for analysis to see if a situation can be 'dangerous' or not and just release an anxious response anyway. This is what happens when people have their first panic attack. This is why panic, or intense anxiety, seemingly comes from 'nowhere'. You must remember that anxiety can occur even out of our control. What's positive though, is that we can control what we do in response to it, in order to turn it off.

Adrenaline & Cortisol

Really super important this: the reason why we feel so scared when we are anxious is because of *hormones* – primarily the powerful chemicals of adrenaline (epinephrine) and cortisol. If you have ever felt that "whoosh" feeling of fear, then this is adrenaline being released and coursing around your bloodstream. If you are someone who constantly feels "on-edge", then this is mostly likely a combination of adrenaline (lower levels) and cortisol.

Adrenaline is such a powerful hormone and the amount of adrenaline we feel is often related to how much we worry or panic. Lots of adrenaline can make our heart rate increase, it can make us feel incredibly tense, it can trigger nausea and also acts as a trigger for our mind to race. It can also make us feel really "spaced out" and, at times, contributes to a feeling of derealisation – this is where we feel detached from our bodies, or experience a sense of unreality. For people with an anxiety disorder, it can also make us feel incredibly confused.

"A lot of people develop panic disorder when they suddenly experience a rush of fear for no reason. This is usually called a panic attack, because the confusion surrounding this sudden rush of adrenaline makes us worry more about it. Our focus can suddenly go inwards and we can begin to 'monitor' ourselves for the signs of imminent disaster, such as experiencing a heart attack, losing our minds, freaking out, collapsing, just to name a few." - Josh

When it comes to understanding our own anxiety better, it is important to acknowledge the profound affect adrenaline and cortisol can have on our minds and bodies. Hormones are the integral part of the 'fight, flight or freeze" response and massively contribute to the following:

- **A change in thoughts**: racing thoughts, finding dangers, over-thinking and over-analysing and believing in the worst-case scenario of a situation.

- **A change in feelings**: feelings of fear, dread, doom and negative anticipation. Feeling like something awful is going to happen.

- **Physical changes**: heart palpitation, derealisation, irritable bowel syndrome, chest pains, muscle tension (all over body), headaches, muscle twitches, dizziness, nausea (and many more).

We like to make anxiety as simple as possible when we work with people. Remember, fear and anxiety mean you have adrenaline and cortisol in your bloodstream. This *feeling* is chemical and, importantly, *internal*. It does not mean the 'disaster' or the worry you have been dwelling on will come true.

The Nervous System

Another really important component of anxiety that we must understand is the role of our *nervous system* when it comes to anxiety, in particular the role of the *autonomic nervous system.* Our nervous system is responsible for both voluntary movement (the voluntary system), but also the internal processes of the body which lie mostly out of our control (the autonomic system).

When working with anxiety, we always focus on the autonomic; this is what we will refer to as the 'nervous system' from now on, for simplicity purposes. Our nervous system is split into two parts:

1. Sympathetic Nervous System

The sympathetic nervous system is responsible for triggering our body's fight, flight or freeze response. It is responsible for triggering the adrenal glands (hello again adrenaline!) and also responsible for altering the function of our vital organs. Anxiety aside, our sympathetic nervous system is engaged every time we are in performance mode, or perhaps under pressure at work, or enduring prolonged stress due to life circumstances. It helps us to perform under stress by providing the necessary bodily changes to accommodate our need. These are the nerves that the famous Dr Claire Weekes suggested get very tired. She suggested that excessive anxiety and worry occurs when our nerves get exhausted – something that we agree with! Ultimately, when stress gets too much, this puts us in a susceptible position to experience anxiety and a misfiring amygdala. Try and think of the sympathetic nervous system as the part that "gets us through stuff!".

2. Parasympathetic Nervous System

The parasympathetic system is the restorative part of our nervous system that is activated when we are resting, eating, enjoying something, experiencing relief and sleeping. This is the part of our nervous system that activates when we lie down after a long day, put the television or radio on, and "switch off for the day". The key information here being that it is activated when we *rest*.

The parasympathetic nervous system acts as a restorative part of our body that helps us to regenerate, process food, helps us to sleep and to give rest to our body's vital organs.

People who are stressed for a long period of time rely on the sympathetic nervous system to get them through the day. However, they really need to find time to activate the parasympathetic system in order to find balance. Ultimately, if we don't have balance, this can lead to excessive anxiety...

The role of stress in disordered anxiety

When working in his practice, or when giving talks to organisations, Josh often draws upon the analogy of a *stress jug*, which is a metaphor for our ability to cope with and absorb stress. He explains that, when we experience stress – in any form – it gets poured into our jug. This includes everyday stress, such as finances, our career, parenting, being a carer, chronic illness, etc. However, it also includes long-term, unprocessed stress such as grief, an unhappy relationship, trauma and emotional turbulence from our past.

Our *stress jug* can handle a lot of stress, hence why the people around us are not continually having panic attacks. We simply do not get sucked into an anxious hole that immobilises us every time we deal with something stressful. However, when stress builds up and that *sympathetic nervous system* gets overused, our *stress jug* can become overwhelmingly full.

When any receptacle is full, we run the risk of it spilling out, or overflowing, and it is at this point we experience excessive anxiety, which can easily develop into an anxiety disorder.

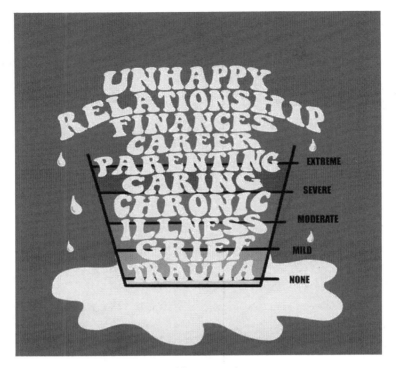

@selfcarevisuals

In summary, when our stress jug overflows, we experience excessive anxiety, which includes panic attacks:

"People often tell me that their acute anxiety seems to 'occur from nowhere'. This is something I used to believe, but actually acute anxiety, which is that flood of adrenaline, along with the racing thoughts, feelings and strange symptoms, occurs because our body simply doesn't want to take on more stress. It's like a warning signal for us to stop. People with disordered anxiety, however, do not stop. They get caught in loops!" – Josh

Here is where understanding the *amygdala* (our lizard brain) is important. When we get overstressed, or overworked, the amygdala gets tricked into thinking we are in actual danger. Remember, the amygdala does not take chances; it activates to save us 'just in case' our life is at risk – remember how you felt when someone startled you, or you jolted awake when you dreamt of falling? Well, the amygdala interprets stress, or our *stress jug* overflowing, as danger in itself. This is why we get that rush of adrenaline and cortisol and feel like something awful is about to happen.

Let us repeat that:

"…the amygdala interprets stress, or our stress jug overflowing, <u>as danger in itself</u>."

This is where excessive and disordered anxiety comes from.

Our stress builds up, either over time, or as a response to trauma, and this fills up the *stress jug*. We overuse our sympathetic nervous system and the amygdala gets tricked into thinking we're in danger. As a result, it releases a lot of fear hormones, such as adrenaline, which make us feel often the intense fear, or feeling on-edge, or the racing thoughts, or the palpitations, nausea, trembling, etc. When we get confused by this, or don't understand what is going on, we can develop a fear of the sensations and worry about what they mean. We can also get sucked into the 'What if?' thoughts that occur as a result of these sudden changes. We can misinterpret symptoms and become frightened. Fear not though, as this is actually a healthy, normal biological response.

In Conversation

Josh: I don't know about you Dean, but learning about the amygdala for me and the psychoeducation about anxiety in general, was so helpful for me to overcome anxiety. And I use it every day when I work with clients. Because if you don't know what's going on, it's very hard to overcome it. But when you know what's going on and you feel like, "Actually, I'm not going insane this is all quite normal." I found that very empowering- I don't know about you?

Dean: I really did, and I've got a small story about it. When I first went to the doctors and I wanted all these answers of why am I feeling the way I am and what is it. They ran the tests. She told me it was anxiety and she prescribed me with a library card for a book. Now you can imagine an anxious 20-year-old lad being prescribed a library book when he thought that obviously something was seriously wrong. I really thought it was like a misjustice, being like I didn't have a clue why she'd done it. So, anyway I went to the library. I got these books about the biology of anxiety and what is happening to me. Looking back on it, it was one of the most useful tools that anyone could have; and that's learning about what you say regarding the psychoeducation behind the anxious response, the anxious symptoms, and just the reason that the body responds like it does when in an anxious state.

Josh: Yes. "Oh, wow there's not actually much wrong with me." This is actually a natural phenomenon. This is really helpful. If my doctor would have told me that straight away- and I don't want to bad mouth my doctor too much because he needs to know a little about a lot - but if my doctor, or someone, or my mental health nurse, would have just told me a lot of this straight away, it would have saved me a lot of bother, and saved me a lot of time and energy.

Dean: I agree with you. However, the anxious brain, do you not think that you would have like automatically wanted to disregard it and thought "no"? Because a lot of people when they get told "It's just anxiety", it's hard to accept it because the anxiety - the anxious response is telling you no, "what if it isn't just anxiety? what if it's anxiety *and* this new problem?"

Josh: True. That is true and probably *my* anxious brain would have done. I know in rare cases, some doctors are clued up about anxiety and they don't just hastily dismiss and throw medication at people, they'll sit and go, "Okay, do you know what anxiety is? You know how it presents?" And just using basically what we said, the *three components of anxiety* in the sense that you know you get these what ifs, you feel on edge, you get all these symptoms because I had no idea; no one told me. I thought the word "anxiety" just meant you're nervous about something- like being nervous about an exam for example - so if someone actually told me what it meant, I think it would save me a lot of bother and I hear this a lot from a lot of my clients. When you make them feel reassured, normal, like they're there's nothing wrong with them, they're not broken, you don't need to fix them, it does a lot of the work. It's like, "Oh I don't need to keep responding to this anxiety like I'm broken."

Dean: I completely agree with you. I can only stress, obviously the natural response of anxiety has been helping humanity since the dawn of time. Without it we wouldn't have been able to evolve as a species. However, today we just don't have the threat we did when we were out hunting and coming across things that can really um probably eat us alive. So, we're-

Josh: I don't know, you grew up in Oldham [Dean laughs], didn't you?

Dean: Yeah, Rochdale.

Josh: Rochdale, oh gosh yeah. I don't know if that's better or worse.

Dean: Yes. I think it's yeah, lineal. [Laughter] However, no, the problem is- well it's not a problem, but the response system reacts to a perceived threat exactly the same it would as a real threat. So, when we're in the office and we get a what-if or we zone in on a feeling that we've got that feels uncomfortable, that perceived threat is going to give the exact same anxious response as if we were in the wild and there was a tiger staring down at us.

Chapter 4

The Symptoms of Anxiety

Featured Artist: @ellamaestatham

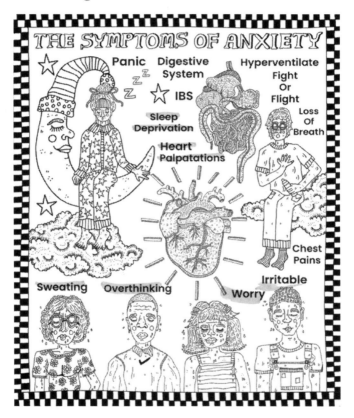

When we were both recovering, we found it really useful to have some of the symptoms of anxiety explained for us. The reason being that anxiety comes with an abundance of intense and confusing symptoms, which can easily lead to more worries that end up on the ever-building worry pile. When working with anxious people, we find it really helpful to apportion strange feelings and sensations to the label of 'anxiety', rather than focussing on each and every symptom and treating it as a worry in itself. In this section we have listed some of the most common symptoms of anxiety, as well as some of the most strange!

Derealisation / Depersonalisation

This symptom can be really scary, initially. It was the trigger for Josh's first panic attack and very common amongst anxiety sufferers. Derealisation can be described as a feeling of unreality, or feeling 'detached' from either ourselves or our surroundings. Derealisation occurs when we just "don't feel right", with our senses being slightly skewed, but we can't quite describe it to others. Here are some of the descriptions of derealisation that we have heard from clients over the years:

- I can hear myself talk but it doesn't feel like me talking.

- It feels like I'm living in a dream world that isn't my reality.

- It feels like I can see myself in third person.

- I just feel really spaced out and not in the room.

- People's faces don't look real, as if they are made of clay.

- It feels like the first sign of me going crazy.

Derealisation and depersonalisation are actually harmless and it is *not* the first sign of you going crazy. It can feel uncomfortable, but when it catches us unawares, it can trigger the anxious response and we may begin to fear it. The reason why we suddenly feel this symptom is a combination of two factors:

1. We stress breathe and slowly hyperventilate

When we are stressed, or anxious, our breathing pattern changes (usually without our awareness). We take in more oxygen than normal and, as a result, our blood oxygen levels increase and with that comes its own symptoms. Stress breathing also includes breathing out less, which means less carbon dioxide leaves the body. This is called hyperventilation and can occur over several days... and not just to someone who's panicking. It can therefore easily go unnoticed. Hyperventilation means there is more oxygen in the blood, which leads to light-headedness, dizziness, numbness and an array of bodily changes. This is part one of why we feel so 'strange' when we experience derealisation.

2. Fight-or-flight

When we are anxious, we are in fight-or-flight mode. Whether we are panicking, or just feeling on edge, this is still some form of fight-or-flight. When in fight-or-flight mode, the body redistributes blood to our major muscle groups in the lower part of our body. It does this to engage us to run faster (away from predators), or to fight* predators.

*Side note: Dean and Josh are big softies and wouldn't fight anyone.

Importantly, as a result of this, this means there is less blood flow in the brain, as well as a shift in blood pressure. This also contributes to the strange feelings of derealisation and detachment. The higher blood oxygen level from over-breathing, combined with the temporarily reduced blood flow in the brain due to fight-or-flight, is why we feel spaced out and "derealised".

Hyperventilating

So a little bit more on this. Another common symptom that occurs when anxious or experiencing panic is hyperventilating. Our breathing may become shallow and restricted as we take in quick short breaths, which, in turn, causes carbon dioxide levels in the blood to decrease. This symptom, like every anxiety symptom, can often come out of nowhere and can be frightening. Unfortunately, an anxious person's natural response to this would be to breath even quicker and shallower, which in turn will increase the anxiety further. Many people who experience this symptom often describe it as a choking or suffocating sensation.

Normally we are not aware of our regular 'normal' breathing. However, when panic and anxiety occur, we can become hypersensitive to our breathing and focus on the fact that we feel breathless or we cannot breathe properly. Our relationship with this thought 'I cannot breathe' can increase our anxiety further causing an anxious person to take in quicker, more shallow breaths.

This reduction in carbon dioxide in the blood can cause many other physical symptoms such as tingling, chest pain, numbness and dry mouth.

Hyperventilation can develop into feelings of dizziness, light headedness and feeling faint. This is due to the narrowing of the blood vessels that supply blood to the brain.

It is worth noting that for some people hyperventilating is rare; it can only occur as an occasional response to panic or fear. Hyperventilating will increase the heart rate and you may feel that your hands and feet are cold - it can also cause feelings of nausea and sickness.

So why does hyperventilating occur?

When we are anxious or feeling stressed, we tend to carry a lot of tension in our body especially our upper body. This can affect the ability of the diaphragm to function efficiently, which in turn puts more pressure onto the breathing muscles. Prolonged overuse of these muscles can lead to breathlessness and as a response to this feeling, an anxious person may then hyperventilate. The main problem with hyperventilating - just like other scary anxiety symptoms - is that the symptom often leads to further anxiety. Often people who deal with this symptom are convinced that there must be some other medical explanation and will disregard that anxiety is at play. Many people who suffer from anxiety and panic will over-breathe even when they think they are relaxed. When an anxious person is hyperventilating, they will often feel that they are not getting enough oxygen into their body, which leads us onto the next symptom:

Struggling to catch breath

Another common symptom of anxiety is when people complain

that they cannot catch their breath. They may also feel like that they can't take a "full breath" or a satiating filling of the lungs. The reason why we have put this symptom third is because it links fittingly with *derealisation* in the sense that this, too, is down to stress breathing, or hyperventilation.

When we take in too much air, the body, very intelligently, steps in to regulate the amount of oxygen in the bloodstream. It does this by preventing us from taking in more oxygen than we need. Basically, if you are often anxious and struggle to catch your breath (with no related health condition), then this is because the body is telling you that you have *too much* oxygen.

Of course, if we don't know this and we are anxious, we may begin to misinterpret this as a sign of us not being able to breathe properly. Unfortunately, we then attempt the opposite of what the body wants us to do; we begin to try and breathe in more! This is why, during panic attacks, some people end up having tingling hands and feet, as well as feeling extremely lightheaded. Fear not though, as the body always brings us back to balance, whether you panic or not.

Remember, panic cannot stop you from breathing!

Heart Palpitations & Flutters

It is absolutely normal for our heart to pound and our *beats per minute* to increase during anxiety. This happens as a result of the adrenaline and cortisol that is released as part of the anxious response. It is also common for our heart to palpitate and flutter during periods of prolonged anxiety. This includes the occurrence of *ectopic beats,* where it feels like our heart is 'skipping a beat' or doubling up on beats. If you do have a concern though, we implore you to check in with your doctor just to make sure and you can then have the appropriate tests.

Digestive System Problems

The symptoms of anxiety can often mimic the symptoms of Irritable Bowel Syndrome (IBS) because, when we are anxious, the body prioritises the threat response over the need to digest and process food. As a result, the digestive tract slows down, which causes several symptoms associated with IBS. These include:

- Stomach bloating

- Acid Reflux (heartburn)

- Diarrhoea

- Constipation

- Stomach Cramps

- Haemorrhoids / Piles

- Trapped Wind

It takes a lot of energy for the body to engage a fight-or-flight response, which can cause the digestive cycle to be put temporarily on hold. This can lead to a build-up of undigested food from the stomach to the colon, which leads to all sorts of bodily changes, such as the release of more stomach acid, the 'flushing' of the digestive tract (diarrhoea) and the 'blockage' that can make us constipated.

Chest Pains

A scary symptom for some is the occurrence of chest pains. These can present in a few ways, usually as short, stabbing pains, a dull ache, or a 'tearing' type of sensations across the chest area. They can be particularly scary when they are experienced alongside heart palpitations, or chest 'flutters', as anxious people can misinterpret this as the sign of an impending heart attack, or an ongoing heart problem.

Chest pains are one of the most common symptoms of anxiety and they usually occur because of posture and muscle tension. When we are anxious, all of our muscles contract in order to compensate for all the adrenaline and cortisol we process as part of fight, flight or freeze. As a result of this, we often hunch forward, push our shoulders and head forwards and the chest absorbs a lot of the muscle tension. When these muscles relax, we notice that the chest feels tense and can often feel painful. Obviously, if you are concerned, get checked over by the doctor just to make sure.

Sweating / Perspiration

Sweating is another common physical symptom of anxiety. Let's look at the reason behind why we sweat when we are feeling panic and anxiety. When our body goes into its fight or flight response, our sympathetic nervous system releases hormones including adrenaline which in turn activates our sweat glands.

One interesting study of brain scans revealed that sniffing someone else's panic induced sweat (as gross as that may sound) lights up areas of the brain that handle emotional and social signals. One theory is that this sweating is an evolved behaviour that makes other brains alert to whatever threat or perceived threat is making us anxious.

Another theory why we sweat has to do with when our ancestors would hunt in the wild and be open to attack from predators. It is believed the sweat would make it easy for us to slip away if anything caught us.

Sweating has a lot of advantages: it will eventually evaporate from the skin cooling the body temperature to prevent elevated internal temperatures. This is not specifically needed for anxiety though, so is seen as more of an annoyance to those experiencing anxiety.

As with all anxiety symptoms, nervous sweating can lead to increased sweating because we may feel self-conscious about it - especially if we are in a social situation. If sweating is a symptom of anxiety this cycle is probably all too familiar for you:

You sweat = You get hypersensitive to the fact you are sweating and the thought 'sticks' in your mind = you sweat more.

Sweating doesn't only occur with anxiety disorders; it can occur with everyday social situations that can make anyone nervous such as:

Public speaking

Making a request

Meeting new people

Job interviews

Being put into an unfamiliar situation

Excessive sweating is known to occur as a primary symptom in as many as 32% of people who have a social anxiety disorder.

Problems with Sleep

There is a huge correlation between lack of sleep or broken sleep and increased anxiety. Excess worry and fear make it harder to fall asleep and stay asleep through the night. Lack of sleep can increase anxiety levels which causes a negative cycle with each aspect fuelling the other.

So, we know anxiety causes lack of sleep, but did you know this? A lot of research has been done on sleep deprivation and it is thought that lack of sleep can be a cause for developing an anxiety disorder. Insomnia and nightmares are listed as common symptoms in general anxiety disorder and post-traumatic stress disorder. As much as one third of the adult population reports difficulty sleeping.

One interesting study by Mellman and Uhde found that compared to healthy subjects, people with panic disorders reported more complaints of 'middle of the night insomnia' and 'late night insomnia', though the two groups did not differ with regards to early night insomnia.

Many people with panic disorder experience occasional sleep panic attacks.

Just like anxiety sleep problems can impact how you function emotionally, mentally and physically. Just the like the old question 'which comes first, the chicken or the egg?' researchers have found that the relationship between sleep problems and anxiety is bidirectional. It's important to note that treating sleep problems without taking steps to manage anxiety is unlikely to have any real lasting impact.

Difficulty concentrating

Having difficulty concentrating or a feeling that your mind goes blank is a common symptom with many anxiety disorders. Anxiety can make us become hyper focused on a thought that appears to be 'stuck' in our mind or a physical sensation we have suddenly become aware of and often distracts us from whatever task we were in the middle of.

Anxiety can also make us focus on irrational thoughts that seem to be spiralling or jumping from one to another. These are caused by your body becoming overly activated to the point where it starts processing all thoughts as rapidly as possible only to end up focusing on nothing at all.

Calling it a lack of concentration is misleading as you *are* concentrating: you are just focusing on the wrong things like the anxiety you are feeling and how it is making you feel. It is very hard to focus on a task at hand when you feel that your mind is trying to make you focus on these uncomfortable thoughts, sensations and feelings.

Many people use distractions to cope with anxiety. For example, you may find yourself checking your phone more when you are in a heightened state of anxiety because you find that checking your phone relaxes you. However, by doing this you could be distracting yourself from the task at hand and it will make it difficult to focus.

And the rest!

Anxiety presents with a lot of symptoms. It is easier to understand if we split them into two categories: mental symptoms and physical symptoms.

Mental symptoms of anxiety can include:

Racing thoughts

Uncontrollable overthinking

Difficulty concentrating

Feelings of dread, panic and impending doom

Feeling irritable

Heightened alertness

Problems with sleep

Change in appetite

Wanting to flee from the situation you are in

Depersonalisation

Derealisation

Physical symptoms of anxiety can include:

Sweating

Heart palpitations/increased heart rate

Hyperventilating

Hot flushes

Shaking

Dry mouth

Dizziness

Nausea and other gastrointestinal issues

Eye floaters

Muscle twitching

Always check with your doctor

Although anxiety is responsible for a myriad of physical symptoms, always check with your doctor if you are concerned, or if the symptoms are prolonged, or seem to be getting worse. It's better to be safe and also to reassure ourselves.

In Conversation

Josh: Okay Dean, I want your top three favorite, spiciest symptoms of anxiety, and I'll give you mine.

Dean: My top three, would definitely have to be the emotional impending doom, so the fear mentioned in the first chapter; so that sense of impending doom; "something seriously is going to go wrong."

Josh: Oh yeah, I hate that. It's so convincing as well, isn't it?

Dean: It really is yeah. And it all almost gives you a sense of terror, doesn't it?

Josh: Yeah, you're just like, "Oh my god", but for me what added to the terror was that my rational brain knew there wasn't really anything wrong, so then I'd worry about why I was worrying. I'd start panicking about why I felt so scared because then I just thought, "well there must be something wrong with my brain." If doom is there, then there must be something happening and only after a while it's like, "Ah it's a trick, it's a false alarm of the brain."

Dean: And I think it's worth noting that if we didn't have that trick, that false alarm, then anxiety wouldn't be doing what its role is which is to convince you that there is a threat and there is a danger. So, that impending doom is exactly what's needed in an anxious response.

Josh: Yeah, looking out for predators and all that. Okay that's number one. What's your other two?

Dean: Number two, it definitely has to be heart palpitations or increased heart rate. I can go back to wearing a Fitbit. I used to do some running, believe it or not [laughter]. You won't believe it at the moment.

Josh: There's no mystery behind that wonderful physique of yours.

Dean: [Laughter] So, yeah, I used to do some running and one thing being anxious and having a Fitbit on is that it's telling you your current heart rate, which was a blessing and also a curse. Because when you're in an anxious moment, I remember being sat in the office at work looking at my Fitbit, and as I looked at it, seeing my heart increase and looking down and then thinking "why is it increasing? All I'm doing is sat here at my computer?" Then the more I thought about it, the more it increased the more other physical symptoms will start to occur.

Josh: Oh yeah? And your third?

Dean: My third one would be...

Josh: You don't need to describe it just what was it that you just didn't like about it?

Dean: Oh, probably sweating you know, and I think it's one that's not discussed a lot. Obviously being in the office having to wear shirts and be presentable and then obviously knowing that I'm anxious and sweating. It can make it uncomfortable the situation you're in because then you can focus on- do you know what I mean? What happens if people are thinking "Why 'am I' just sitting sweating my clothes off?" [Laughter]

Josh: Brilliant. Brilliant. Mine were- my worst one for me was derealization, the sense of detachment used to freak me out. I thought that was the first sign of my brain breaking or something. The other one was chest pain.

Dean: Yeah.

Josh: You know and when you have chest pain and palpitations. I mean, your anxious brain just goes to one place, doesn't it?

Dean: Yes.

Josh: Oh my god, there's something wrong with my heart... and the last one that really took me long time to overcome was struggling to catch my breath. I always thought, "Oh my gosh I can't breathe. I can't catch my breath. Obviously now I know it's because we breathed too much throughout the day but...

Dean: Yes.

Josh: And they were my three spiciest ones. But obviously there's loads of them. I must have experienced over 30 symptoms of anxiety.

Dean: Just going back to the chest pains, how would you explain that? Was it like a sharp pain for you or was it like a crushing pain?

Josh: Multiple, crushing, stretching, stabbing pains. There are different types of pain you know because the muscles are constantly contracting and expanding, contracting and expanding, and because their chest muscles are so big - well mine are anyway because I'm really hench [laughs].

Chapter 5

Anxiety is a Threat Response

Featured Artist: @crazyheadcomics

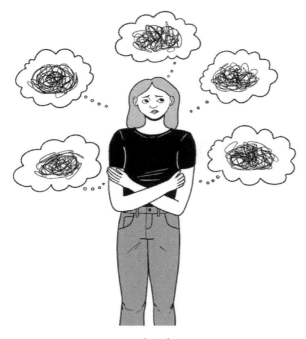

@crazyheadcomics

We think it is really helpful to describe anxiety as a threat response when it comes to learning about anxiety and overcoming it. To put it simply, an excessive anxiety problem is when our threat response *misfires* at times when we don't want it to. Also, and perhaps most importantly, disordered anxiety occurs when our threat response is triggered after it has been unintentionally *conditioned* to. For example, many people with panic disorder have an amygdala that has been conditioned to trigger at the first signs of panic, such as shortness of breath, derealisation, dizziness, palpitations, etc. This also applies to social anxiety, where our amygdala can be triggered by people, or even agoraphobia, where our threat response can be triggered by even the thought of going outside.

You Are Not Broken

A common belief that people with anxiety often subscribe to is the belief that they are in some way 'broken'. This is *simply not true* and we will explain why. Anxious thoughts and vivid imaginations are actually signs of intelligence; they form part of our rationalisation process, which is when the brain scans through all the potential scenarios and their consequences. For example, before we attempt to cross a road, it is helpful to imagine that we may be struck by a moving vehicle, as it would influence us to look in both directions before stepping out. Similarly, we may be tempted to cut through a park at night, only to avoid it because of some suspicious looking people hanging out in the shadows. The thought of being assaulted may actually keep us safe by influencing our decision to take a safer walk home.

Unfortunately, this influencing process can become entangled in our day to day lives and our brains can start to "figure out" the worst-case scenarios of situations where we are categorically safe! When the threat response triggers, this engages the mind to scan the situation and provide all the potential dangers that could occur. This is why people with health anxiety suddenly believe that a headache could suddenly be a brain tumour, or heart palpitations could be the sign of heart failure. Similarly, people who panic misinterpret normal signs of fight or flight as the firsts step towards insanity or losing control. It is the *threat response* that triggers this rationalisation process when it simply isn't needed - the person with social anxiety suddenly misinterprets a facial expression as the sign of rejection, or the person with GAD thinks that the email from their boss is to summon them to a meeting where they will be fired.

We must also remember that when our amygdala misfires, it also creates the *feelings* and *sensations* that come with the fight, flight or freeze response. This adds an extra layer to anxious suffering and provides a mental lens that suddenly makes our thoughts *feel* a bit more real. We don't react emotionally to the vast majority of our thoughts, but if our threat response has been triggered, and we are experiencing the effects of adrenaline and cortisol, then suddenly this can magnify the intensity of scary thoughts. For example, on a calm morning we can imagine weird thoughts, such as "what if I go insane?" and they don't seem to affect us. However, that same thought can appear and feel more terrifying if the threat response has already been triggered.

You must remember that, just because your threat response has been triggered, this does not mean you are broken in any way. Excessive anxiety is a *condition,* which by its very definition means that it can be changed to an alternate state. Just because your amygdala and threat response are misfiring and you're dealing with lots of adrenaline does not mean you are permanently ill. You can and will recover.

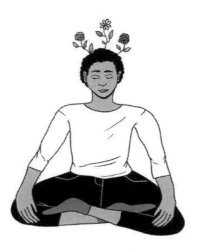

@crazyheadcomics

Overcoming Anxiety is Turning Off the Threat Response

In simple terms, overcoming an anxiety condition is when we successfully manage to turn off the threat response during times when we do not need it. You must remember that anxiety cannot be completely eradicated – it is a normal, essential and healthy function of our minds and bodies. We need the threat response to live! It is extremely helpful and has probably saved our lives countless times in the past, but over time we meet it with no gratitude, as we undoubtedly start to resent it when we live each day with it unnecessarily.

When Josh works with anxious clients at The Panic Room and asks them what they would like to get from therapy, he often hears statements like, "I just want to feel like my normal self again" and "I just want to stop feeling like this!" In essence, what these clients are actually requesting is:

"I would like to turn off my body's threat system. It is scary and uncomfortable."

We really hope you join us in our conceptualisation of anxiety being a threat response. All that fear, uncertainty, racing thoughts, physical symptoms, apprehension, catastrophe-based beliefs and monitoring are all part of the same response.

When looking at the neurobiology of this threat response, it is really important to understand how we can interact with the amygdala in order to switch it off. We cannot, however, control the amygdala ourselves, but we can heavily influence its decision to turn the threat response on and off. Ultimately, when the amygdala decides there is no danger, it switches off. This is when we stop experiencing the feelings and sensations associated with adrenaline and cortisol and return to feeling calm and "normal". When we no longer feel anxious, this is when the amygdala has switched off!

Importantly, we must remember that we cannot talk to the threat response: words mean nothing to it. This is because the amygdala is only wired to our thinking brains in *one direction*, meaning that the amygdala can send signals to our thinking brain, but we are unable to send information back to it. This is why talking to your anxiety doesn't really work. Think about it, how many times have you tried to 'talk yourself down' or tell the anxiety 'to go away', or even use words to convince yourself? It doesn't work for this very reason.

However, what *does* work is when we *show* the amygdala using our senses. By facing fear – or what the amygdala defines as 'danger' – we can actively begin to turn off the anxious response, so that it doesn't trigger in the future and we can begin to live our normal lives again. This does require being a bit courageous, but you will be being so in the knowledge that you are safe.

The Purpose of the Threat Response

Have you ever wondered why you feel on edge a lot? Feeling on edge is like a mild form of the threat response. When we feel on edge our attention is usually heightened and we're on hyper-alert like a meerkat. As our senses sharpen, our thoughts become more detailed and more dangerous. We can become *hypervigilant*. But, what's the purpose of that? Our friend, the meerkat, needs this hypervigilance so that he can flee from an approaching jackal (or stick up his fists if he's feeling that brave). But what has that got to do with us sitting at home, feeling on edge as the Wi-Fi fails to work during an important business meeting held online? In day-to-day life, what's the point of it?

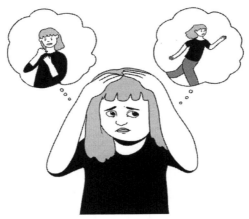

@crazyheadcomics

71

To greater understand the purpose of this threat response, we must understand it *biologically*. We need to take a look at two important hormones: cortisol and adrenaline. Although both of these hormones play an extremely important role in the threat response, we will primarily focus on cortisol to help us understand it from a biological standpoint. Cortisol is a hormone that we call the 'stress hormone'. It is released from the adrenal gland, the same place that releases adrenaline. If we're calling this the 'stress hormone' we might sit there and wonder, "What is the purpose of releasing cortisol when I'm trying to eat my bowl of Weetabix in the morning?" We should feel comfortable in times like these when we're simply moving through our daily routines. So, what's the purpose of releasing cortisol when we're not in any *immediate* danger? Let's take a look…

When we are stressed in our minds and bodies, we can easily get confused and perceive that we are under threat. Yet, it is when we are under *immediate* threat that we release the hormone adrenaline. Adrenaline is what gives us that boost of energy to make us feel as though we can wrestle with bears or at least out-run them despite never having run a yard in our lives. When adrenaline kicks in we take *immediate* action, whether that be defending ourselves (fight) or fleeing the scene (flight). If a predator comes after you, it's the adrenaline that you will need. However, we've only got limited amounts of this hormone. So if we're walking around in our day-to-day lives using up all of our adrenaline, what's going to happen when that bear wanders around the corner and we suddenly need to take action? We've run out of adrenaline so we can't fight back and we can't run either. Luckily there is a middle man and that middle man, is *cortisol.*

Where cortisol is concerned, we can have more of it. When this cortisol runs through our bodies we can stay in a half-threat, half-normal mode, which is where the sensation of feeling on edge comes into play. You can still function but you don't necessarily feel relaxed: this is cortisol. Cortisol keeps us in this state of high alert so that when we do find ourselves under threat, we can quickly engage with adrenaline when we need it.

Picture this scene. We are back on the planes of the Serengeti thousands of years ago and there are predators everywhere. Imagine lions, hyenas, and cheetahs roaming in every direction. Cortisol, in this instance, is keeping us on high alert. This is really important in this scenario because, as humans, we're going to do a pretty terrible job when face to face with a lion. We can't fight it and we can't run away from it. The likes of Usain Bolt could give it a good go but even his superhuman speed is unlikely to save him here. So, what's the point? Cortisol helps us maintain this state of high alert, which is crucial to our survival in the Serengeti because what this stress hormone does is allow us to *see the predator coming.* We don't want to wait until it is right on top of us to trigger the threat response; in these conditions we want to remain extra vigilant so that we can mitigate risk and avoid danger. Cortisol in effect has saved our lives *in advance* by making us aware of what is going on around us. Perhaps we hear a rustle in the trees and wisely decide to steer clear, which in turn could keep us safe. We might think, "There is a noise among those trees... I don't know what it could be but it might be a predator... I'm not going to aimlessly walk among the overgrowth and into a potentially dangerous situation... better keep away". This is thanks to cortisol.

Of course, cortisol is great if you find yourself in the Serengeti. Yet our threat response gets confused because in day-to-day life we are looking for predators that aren't there. The reason it benefits to understand what cortisol is and how it functions within this threat response is so that we *don't engage with it.* If we have cortisol running through our bodies and we entertain it, we might sit there in an otherwise safe environment and think to ourselves, "What if they think I'm ridiculous or what if I throw up in front of everyone or what if... what if... what if..." It's an incredible waste of our energy that could be far better used elsewhere. We get caught up thinking that these messages are real in our daily lives but they are not real messages.

For example, if you have social anxiety and you're worrying about a party two weeks in advance or you have an appraisal due from work that you are fixating on, then that is a prime example of living in a state of high alert. You might ruminate, "What if they say that..." or "What if that does happen..." When we listen to it we keep the stress response on when it doesn't need to be. In turn, this only perpetuates our stress surrounding the situation.

In the modern-day, our stress response tries to apply itself to modern things and that's where we get confused. It's quicker to engage in fight or flight if you're already half in it, making it quicker and easier for the adrenaline to kick in and help us flee before anything really bad happens. In reality, the dangers we face in everyday life aren't real dangers. Nothing really bad is likely to happen. Consider this, have you ever watched a scary movie that has left you feeling on edge only for your partner to touch your arm afterward and have you jump out of your skin? This is the exact same thing. The cortisol is keeping you in a state of high alert so that the adrenaline is in easy reach when it's needed.

So, what's the purpose of the threat response? It can save us *in advance*. Quite frankly, we're not great at fighting and we're not great at running, so it's there to help us avoid having to do either of these things: conserving our adrenaline, but not allowing us to relax. If we were in the Serengeti, we could truly appreciate the biology and necessity for this cortisol threat response.

In Conversation

Josh: What really interested me Dean was the different roles of the anxious chemicals. So, I didn't know this for ages, but cortisol is what keeps us on edge. And that's because, you know, if we're on the Serengeti and we're looking for predators, you know we can't fight or run away from a lion because we're rubbish at it, but the cortisol helps to keep us on edge, so we can see them coming from a mile away. This is the exact same response that we have now. Annoyingly, we don't need cortisol to see our annoying boss coming from a mile away, we don't need cortisol to anticipate an email coming in to threaten us. But also, the role of adrenaline when that perceived danger actually occurs appears like 'bam!'. And that's suddenly when we feel the terror - the fear, the "oh my gosh, something bad's going to happen", and the racing heart and the imminent doom. And I just thought it was really interesting, because as a threat response it makes sense. I can see that making sense hundreds and thousands of years ago, it's just quite difficult to get our head around now. Do you see any positives in having that threat response now?

Dean: It all depends on the situation, because obviously anxiety gets a bad rep, but it's what keeps us safe in situations. So, anxiety is obviously still needed in certain situations which [do you know what I mean?], could be life-threatening. So, if you think about it, if we didn't have it we'd be wandering around care-free...

Josh: Just walking into traffic [laughs].

Dean: Yeah, you need that rush to almost like make your reactions like go super quick? So, you don't get run over.

Josh: I can imagine socially as well - you don't want to go up to the biggest, toughest person and just say what you think, you need anxiety to shut you up.

Dean: [Laughter] Yeah 100%.

Josh- "Your haircut's really offensive. Oops- run!"

Dean: But sat in the office and having a rush of these strong chemicals is where the downside can be because yeah, it's just an intense feeling. And almost like when someone has an espresso coffee, that feeling of the increased heart rate almost mimics the anxiety response, doesn't it? So, I suppose being sat in the office and having this rush of chemicals, it can obviously be very scary.

Chapter 6

Exposure (Done Right)

Featured artist: @justgirlproject

Illustrator: @eriicalewiis

The way we begin to start turning off anxiety, or our 'threat response', is to start practising exposure. Exposure therapy is a tried and tested approach to turning off disordered and phobic anxiety and was pioneered by great behaviourists such as Joseph Wolpe, Stanley Rachman and Ivan Pavlov. At the core of exposure therapy is the concept of *systematic desensitisation,* which is a therapeutic technique in which we use exposure to desensitise ourselves to our anxiety and our *fear* of anxiety. You may have heard of exposure before, or even 'tried it' for yourself, but to no avail. However, exposure therapy is only effective when done correctly. We have set out this chapter to explain it for you in ways that we used for ourselves when setting out towards recovery.

"Exposure therapy is the number one therapy that helped me overcome panic disorder and begin to live a life that I was more familiar with - pre-panic disorder Dean. It sounds crazy right, expose yourself to the fear that is making you anxious, you're telling me I must go to the places I know that I will feel heightened levels of anxiety and most likely will have a panic attack, this is how I am going to overcome the anxiety and panic? Yes! Even though our minds are trying to convince us that we should take all necessary steps to avoid any past triggering situations. What this is doing is conditioning the fear, increasing the intensity and duration of your panic disorder. This often leads to further mental health conditions developing such as specific phobias and agoraphobia, as you try and do everything to avoid what is causing the anxiety." - Dean

In the previous chapter, we discussed that anxiety is better conceptualised as a 'threat response', which is what it literally is in a biological sense. If you find yourself in a state of worry, with physical symptoms, racing thoughts, a sense of doom, dread and fear and a fixation on how you feel, then this, in simple terms, is the body's threat response. I think we would be stating the obvious when we ask "wouldn't it be nice to turn off the threat response?" Well this is the perspective we need to look at it from.

Exposure is not "well just go and do it!" Too many people fall into this trap of misbelieving that exposure is just a simplified, almost dismissive solution to overcoming anxiety. This simply is not true. Exposure and psychoeducation combined is an incredibly effective arsenal to utilise in challenging and overcoming anxiety, as well as knowing all the *do's* and *do nots.*

"I remember that I kept trying to force myself into situations to challenge the anxiety, but it never went away. Looking back, I realised I was "white-knuckling" my way through everything. I would always count down to the moment I could start retreating or doing my own version of 'escaping' the situation, whether it was literally escaping, or emotionally escaping using alcohol." – Josh

When we know why we are 'doing exposure', backed up with the knowledge and reassurance that we are *safe* enough to do it, then that's when the real change happens! We begin a process of rewiring the brain; we then begin to notice that we can tolerate anxious feelings and sensations. This then leads to confidence in our ability to cope and speeds up the recovery process. Ultimately, the goal is to get to a place where we *wilfully* go towards what makes us anxious, knowing how uncomfortable it will make us feel, then *wilfully* tolerate the thoughts, feelings and sensations. Once we learn that nothing 'bad' happens, and that we can actually tolerate it, both we and the amygdala decide that anxiety itself is no longer a danger.

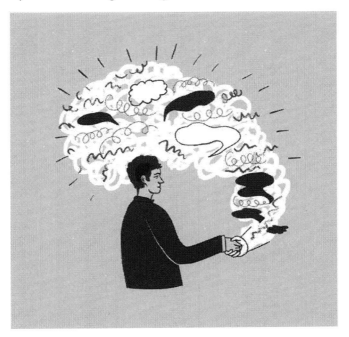

@justgirlproject @eriicalewiis

Secondary Fear

The reason why exposure works effectively for anxiety is twofold: the first being that it turns off the amygdala in situations where we don't need it and the second being that we unknowingly conquer a *phobia*. This phobia being a fear of our own anxious response, also known as *secondary fear*. Anxiety can be uncomfortable and makes us feel scared, but it is something that everyone experiences; it is a healthy and necessary bodily response. However, people with excessive anxiety often develop secondary fear. Here are some examples of common statements from people with secondary fear:

- Why am I so anxious? What does this mean?

- I'm panicking about *why* I'm panicking.

- I avoid doing things *just in case* I get anxious.

- I hope I don't have a panic attack today.

- Is this sensation the first sign of anxiety?

- Do I still feel this derealisation?

- I hope my pulse or heart rate doesn't increase.

- I check to see if I'm anxious when I wake up.

- I just want to feel like my normal self again.

Part of recovery is redefining our relationship with our fear response. It's interesting to reflect on people's relationships with their own fear response, especially when you consider the existence of horror movies, escape rooms and theme parks. Some people actually enjoy evoking the fear response because of the 'rush' it provides – people more colloquially known as 'adrenaline junkies'. This is why people go to watch a scary movie, or queue to be thrown around in the air on a rollercoaster, or pay to experience jump scares. Their relationship with the anxious response is a positive one, helped by the fact that this belief is built upon a foundation of safety.

This is where exposure helps us in the sense that not only do we turn off anxiety in the long run, but we also challenge the phobia, or fear, of anxiety itself, by practising being with it when it arises. The more that we practise this, the easier it becomes, but we must look at how we practise it in order for it to be effective.

Safety Behaviours ("Just in case…")

The biggest hurdle to overcome when practising exposure is the use of *safety behaviours*. Safety behaviours may seem helpful because they reduce anxiety in the short term, however they can become a problem because they keep anxiety going in the long-term. Why is this? Safety behaviours stop us from facing our fears directly and from seeing our fears for what they are Instead they reinforce the notion that 'I must do this certain behaviour in order to stay safe'. This continues the fear of the situation that is causing us anxiety. This is when we make choices and behave in a way that convinces us we are preventing a potential disaster from happening. You know you are engaging in safety behaviours when you do something "just in case" something bad happens. Here are some examples of some common safety behaviours:

- I will go for a walk but I won't go far from home just in case I panic.

- I will attend the meeting, but sit near the door so I can escape if I need to.

- I will attend the party, but I'll stay by my partner's side just in case.

- I will go on holiday, but not without my herbal remedies and tinctures. I will also research nearby hospitals.

- Every time I get a new symptom, I will google it.

- I will walk to work instead of getting transport, just in case I feel trapped.

- I will avoid the highway just in case I panic at the wheel.

- I will always have a safe zone, or safe person, to be near just in case I feel anxiety.

If any of these resonate with you, then it is helpful to label these as *safety behaviours*. When we were recovering, we found it helpful to categorise safety behaviours in two ways:

1 Absolute Avoidance

This is when we categorically avoid doing things for the fear of how we will feel, or for the fear that we may lose control in some way. This applies to people who find it difficult leaving the house, going on vacation, going to new places, meeting new people, or venturing into a new profession.

Remember, to the brain, *avoidance* is the ultimate safety behaviour. The anxious mind wants as close to 100% reassurance that the 'catastrophe' that we fear won't happen. The closest thing we can get to guaranteeing this is by avoiding it as best we can. For example, "what if I panic at the airport?" can be remedied by "well I can't panic at the airport if I don't go!"

It is absolutely imperative to remember that the sole purpose of fight-or-flight is to make you avoid; this threat response wants to keep you safe. However, with disordered anxiety, there isn't actually an identifiable trigger, so implementing safety behaviours in response to extremely unlikely *What if?* thoughts just confuses the anxious brain and puts us into bad habits. *Recovery starts with challenging absolute avoidance.*

2 Micro-avoidance

This is the very sneaky version of avoidance. Have you ever been brave enough to do something you have been avoiding, but it didn't help you overcome the fear? So you still returned home fearing the situation again and again? On most occasions, this is because the brain thought we only got through the event because of a false comfort we brought to exposure, or that we tried to "white knuckle" our way through a scary situation. Here are some examples of micro-avoidances, or 'white-knuckling':

- I'm going to go out, but not without my bag of essential survival supplies, such as water and remedies.

- I'm going to go to the movies, but I'm going to sit on the end of the row.

- I attended the party, but I always stayed near the door.

- I sat through the meeting, but I kept checking the clock and counting down the minutes until I could leave.

- I drove on the highway, but only stayed in the slow lane.

- I climbed the mountain, but only managed it because I was with my wife.

- I managed to buy the groceries, but thankfully I had my smartphone just in case of an emergency.

- I went on vacation, but reassured myself that as each day went by I was a day closer to going home.

We did this for years. We used to "white knuckle" our way through situations, but it was all pivoted on the belief that we could return to our safe spaces. We were getting it all wrong. The whole purpose of exposure is to show the threat response that feeling anxious is ok and not a fear in itself. However, if you think about it, how can challenging exposure be anything to be praised for if we do it with safety items, safe people, or just end up clock-watching? All the brain learns is that we only 'survived' the experience because we could get out of it as soon as possible.

We were still behaving out of fear, so the brain still thinks it is something to be feared.

We can become too reliant on the safety behaviours and thereby more anxious if we are unable to use that particular safety prop. We may thank the safety prop/behaviour for keeping us from feeling anxious. However, we would never know how we would have *truly* coped in the same situation without the safety behaviour, so we continue relying on them and embed our dependence upon them.

Ask yourself: Who is getting the praise here? Is it me for being brave? Or my bag of micro-avoidances and safety behaviours?

Graded Exposure vs Flooding

Now there's two ways of challenging anxiety and that's taking a *graded* approach, or by jumping straight in. We mostly recommend taking a graded approach to challenging the anxious response, so this requires little steps and manageable goals. For example, if our goal is to go to the mall by ourselves, then perhaps try to go to the mall and walk in for 5 minutes, then allow yourself to leave. Then increase the exposure time at each attempt. This can slowly teach the amygdala that the mall is safe. This principle applies to most phobic anxieties. Most therapists will use a graded approach, starting off with mildly feared stimuli and working up to more feared stimuli. This is usually set out in a 'fears hierarchy' and usually higher levels of stimuli are not attempted until lower levels have been overcome.

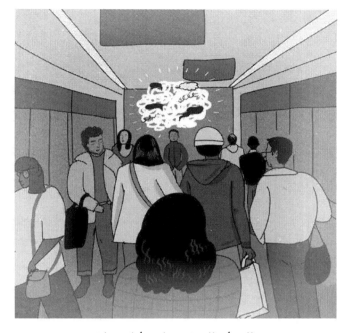

@justgirlproject @eriicalewiis

However, some therapists use a method called *flooding*, in which the most difficult stimuli are introduced right from the beginning of the therapy. Scientifically both methods are deemed equally successful, however clients and therapists tend to use the graded approach because of the personal comfort level. So, if you want to and feel motivated, just go for it! Go and feel anxious and 'flood' yourself with adrenaline in the knowledge that you know it cannot harm you. The feelings will be intense, but they pass relatively quickly. This kind of exposure is highly effective, but we understand why we would choose not to as it can feel quite intense and overwhelming. This is why we can always practise graded exposure, too!

Types of Exposure in CBT

In vivo vs Imaginal

In vivo refers to the real-world exposure to the feared stimuli, however sometimes this exposure is not possible. For example, if a client is suffering from PTSD, due to witnessing explosions in the army, or perhaps they are survivors of sexual abuse, then the triggers cannot be accessed or replicated for obvious reasons.

In these certain cases *imaginal* exposure can be useful. The client is asked to vividly imagine and describe the sights and sounds they would have heard but describe them in present tense terms and also describe what their thoughts and feelings are. ***This work is best done with a trained therapist!***

Interestingly, with technology advancing at a rapid rate, we have seen the introduction of Virtual Reality Exposure Therapy. Clients are immersed into a virtual world to enable them to confront their fears. Preliminary data suggests this form of exposure is effective.

Internal v External

Exposure therapy can target internal and external cues. Some examples of exposure to *external* cues include a snake phobia, or a fear of heights. Exposure work in this case would be learning to train the threat response to turn off by working with snakes and heights, at either a graded level, or by flooding.

However, we understand that a lot of anxiety is *internal*. In CBT, this is called *interoceptive exposure* and this is helpful for people who are frightened of their own anxious sensations. An example of interoceptive exposure would be to run on the spot to increase their heart rate in order to familiarise themselves to the fast heart sensation that they may experience during a panic attack. If you suffer from general anxiety disorder, you may be asked to purposefully induce worrisome thoughts. With a therapist, a client with PTSD can revisit memories and a person with OCD can intentionally evoke intrusive thoughts.

Early exposure therapy used to include relaxation techniques as well as the exposure to certain stimuli. However, after many studies looking into the success of this method it was concluded that it is the 'exposure' rather than the 'relaxation' that gets the results. For years we tried to fix our anxiety by relaxing, but now we understand that relaxing comes *after* we address the problem of turning off the threat response. In fact, in some people - especially those with a panic disorder - relaxation techniques can have a detrimental effect, because the person is not being induced to the physical sensations of the panic attack thus continuing the fear of the physical symptoms panic attacks can produce. According to Dr Sally Winston and Dr Martin Seif, this is called *panicogenic relaxation.*

Dean overcame panic disorder by flooded exposure therapy. His panic attacks would occur in shopping malls. So, to overcome the panic disorder, he would put himself in the middle of a shopping mall and induce the panic response. Instead of leaving the shopping mall, he would continue to walk around and the anxiety and panic would increase. Did he find this scary? Yes, totally! However, each time he did this he would notice that the anxiety levels would decrease a little and the length of time he was anxious would also decrease.

Over time, he was retraining his brain and telling the threat response that the shopping mall was not a dangerous place. It never was before his panic disorder; the only reason it became a trigger was because this was the first place he had a panic attack. Dean had never experienced anything like a panic attack before in his life, so his brain instantly associated the shopping mall with fear. During the worst part of the panic disorder, Dean would feel himself getting anxious around one hour before getting to the shopping mall. Just the thought of going shopping would start to induce an anxious response. The journey to the shopping mall would consist of his palms getting sweaty and his heart rate starting to increase way before he had stepped foot in the shop. This anticipatory anxiety calmed the more he practised and it also helped that he grew in confidence.

Exposure if we are just anxious sat at home

Let's consider what we do if we just get anxious at home, or at work, or in places that we go to frequently and don't avoid. Perhaps our anxiety troubles occur when we are at home just trying to do 'normal' things, such as house chores, running a bath or watching tv. If this is the case, then we can still practise exposure and we can do it very effectively. Being anxious at home is usually prevalent in people with Generalised Anxiety Disorder (GAD) and Panic Disorder. Either way, this is very common and absolutely fine to work with.

Exposure at home happens when we practise sitting, or standing, with anxious feelings, but at the same time, we commit to doing what we would usually be doing if we weren't anxious. Let's rephrase this:

Exposure is when we practise being anxious, whilst continuing to do what we would usually do.

We stress this because a lot of people who experience anxiety at home often check in with their anxiety, monitor it, try to fight it, or even try to fully distract themselves from it. All these responses actually tell the amygdala that feeling anxious itself is something to be concerned about, so we end up in thought/feeling /behaviour loops.

Exposure happens when we say "ok, I'm feeling anxious, but here's a chance to teach my brain that I can still do what I would usually do, but allow anxiety to be there." It's as if we are temporarily accepting the anxiety, but putting all of our effort into our *behaviour*. If we reframe anxiety in this way, we can start to make progress, which ends up in us convincing the threat response to turn off. We'll discuss and outline this further in the next chapter, *Cultivating a New Attitude.*

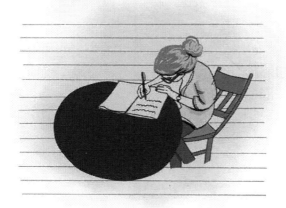

@justgirlproject @eriicalewiis

If you do wish to do something in response to it, in order to demystify the anxiety, then Dean suggests something helpful:

"How do we use exposure therapy when we're feeling anxious all the time, even whilst sitting down at a desk or even at home watching tv? Writing exposure is a CBT method that is used in these situations. People can sit down and write out their irrational thoughts and fears and label how likely they are to come true. The act of taking the irrational thought away from the mind to a piece of paper, taking it from the internal to the external, can have a powerful impact on reducing anxiety. Also, just by sitting through the anxiety and by labelling that you are anxious and for a certain time you will feel uncomfortable, but you know what this feeling is. It is anxiety and it is temporary; it too shall pass like it did in the past and like it will if it arises in the future." – Dean

In Conversation

Dean: So, exposure therapy was the number one part of therapy for me. I used it more in a self-help way to help me overcome the panic disorder. So, as we know there's two different types of exposure therapy from what I know which is gradual and flooded. I use the flooded technique...

Josh: Oof.

Dean: Yeah, I know.

Josh: I used gradual, so fair play.

Dean: The research and science behind it says that, when someone goes to a therapist, they tend to go with the gradual aspect. However, when you put gradual and flooded exposure next to each other, the results tend to be the same. So, I think it's just like on an individual basis, but for myself I preferred flooded exposure - literally putting myself in the middle of the situation. So, I knew that I'd get anxious in the middle of a shopping center. So, what would I do? I'd drive to the shopping center purposely, even though I didn't need a new pair of socks, and I'd put myself in the sock section and let the anxiety come and feel everything that anxiety had to show?

Josh: Did you find that easy?

Dean: I didn't, no. The first time it was terrifying just driving up to the shopping center. I was already feeling anxious, never mind getting out the car and getting into it. After doing it the first time I think I probably went home and I can remember thinking it was a total disaster and I was never going to overcome a panic disorder and this was me, right? And I'm sure you've heard this and you probably felt it yourself Josh, you feel that you're trapped. You don't feel that there's light at the end of the tunnel. You feel that you're isolated and you almost- the brain almost like concludes that, "Yeah this is me and this is how I'm going to have to live my life." However, I kept doing it. I kept persisting and over time I gradually started to see that the anxious response became less intense. I kept putting myself in the situation and I got comfortable with the uncomfortable feeling, if you know what I mean?

Josh: Yeah. Oh, that's brilliant. I mean, that reminds me of when I did it gradually a little bit at a time with certain things. Some things I jumped straight in and with other things I just I built up to it. It just depends what feels right. Both are as effective as one another, so I say to my clients, "You know you choose one or the other and just because you're doing one thing instead of the other, it still means you can get to the same place." For me though, I remember when I was doing my exposure and I did it for a while, but I used to white knuckle and use safety behaviors a bit too much. And I used to get really frustrated, but then I just thought "well you know what, take it to therapy, Josh." And then my therapist would be like, "Alright okay this is what's happening. Actually, you can do it again, but try it without the safety behaviors a little bit at a time." So, actually there's always a positive to take from it.

Dean: And I think you almost see on social media as well these short hacks which aren't actually helpful, like how to use sensory safety behaviors in response to your anxiety. Now sometimes- I'm in two minds. I don't know how you think Josh. I think they can do more harm than good; however, obviously in the situation it might reduce the anxiety there and then. But I don't think it's looking at the overall anxiety disorder. It is not going to be helpful over the long term, is it?

Josh: No. I think one of my most interesting parts of exposure was practising something called "Interoceptive Exposure". So, I used to get really scared of feeling dizzy, so then I'd purposely make myself dizzy and practice tolerating anxiety. I used to be scared of feeling spaced out, so I deliberately hyperventilated to make myself feel spaced out and lightheaded to practice wilful tolerance. I used do things like do press-ups so my chest would ache, so that I could get used to my chest hurting whenever it happened, and so forth and so forth.

Dean: Yeah. Have you ever had a like positive- have you used that in a therapy setting before?

Josh: Oh loads.

Dean: So, I've heard some really good responses on it.

Josh: I've marched clients up and down stairs, so their heart rates increase.

Dean: Yeah.

Josh: You know not physically marched, although that's something I should consider [laughs]

Chapter 7

Cultivating a New Attitude

Featured Artist: @aprilhillwriting

One of the biggest stumbling blocks in anxious recovery is the negative perspective that we view our anxiety from, as well as the way we speak to ourselves when trying to overcome it. The person who approaches tackling anxiety with an attitude of self-forgiveness, compassion and patience, will be the person who gets their life back on track again. Whereas the person who is highly self-critical, who sees anxiety as a sign of failure, then blames themselves for being anxious, will be the one wrestling with it for a little while longer. Cultivating a new, healthier attitude is very important when it comes to anxious recovery.

"There is absolutely no point in challenging anxiety if we are being critical of ourselves." - Josh

We know the psychoeducation side of anxiety now, so let's develop a stronger understanding of how our inner dialogue can affect things, as well as our beliefs around what success actually means. It is imperative that we do not see ourselves as victims, or people that are terminally ill, but as people who are just a bit stuck in a cycle which we can break free from when we attempt to do so correctly. We both passionately believe that everyone can break free from the nasty cycle of anxiety.

The reason why being self-critical does not work is because criticism stimulates the stress response. Think about it, if we followed you around all day – from the moment you woke up – and criticised you for avoiding, criticised you for being anxious, pointed out that you didn't feel yourself and happy, reminded you that you don't feel like your old self, or the people around you, this would be incredibly stressful. The impact of us constantly reminding you and telling you that anxiety has got you and that you're not how you "should" be would have a huge emotional impact. Now imagine the impact that would have if you were saying it to yourself; these critical voices not coming from two strangers, but from within your own mind. This is why perspective is hugely important.

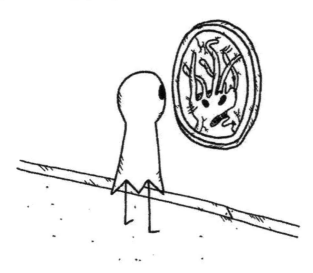

@aprilhillwriting

See Anxiety as a Spectrum, Not Binary

When in his practice, Josh always invites clients to rate their current anxiety on a scale from 1 to 10. This means the anxiety that they are feeling in that very moment. This is important, because anxiety always presents itself at varying levels. You can be experiencing low-level anxiety, where you feel on-edge and unable to relax, or you could be in a panic, which would put you higher up on the scale. Wherever you are on the scale, this is ok.

Too many anxious people fall into the unhelpful thought trap of thinking anxiety is either "here" or "not here" without considering what is happening from a more accurate perspective. Sometimes we can live with low-level anxiety, whereas other times it can feel quite acute. Knowing that anxiety never remains a constant is a helpful thing to know. It really helps with recovery, too. Rather than judging our recovery on whether anxiety is there or not, it helps to break it down into smaller units of measurement. For example, you may walk into a shopping mall with anxiety at a 9 on your anxiety scale, then on leaving it may be a 5. This is some outstanding exposure work and puts you well on the way to recovery. It also means you have successfully lowered your anxiety! Ok, so it may not be ideal or our end goal, but it's a great leap in the right direction. However, self-critical people may perceive this as a failure and we find this heart-breaking.

Start getting into the habit of really getting to know your anxiety levels. If you can notice that your anxiety has come down significantly, or even that it increases as you get closer to a trigger, then this is good mindful observation.

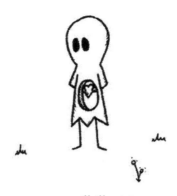

@aprilhillwriting

It'll help you be able to detach from the feelings when practising exposure, or just trying to do something whilst anxiety is present. After all, you needn't avoid doing anything if you're anxious. You're more than capable of doing anything whilst that threat response is firing off. If you can do an activity and leave it feeling less anxious than when you began it, then you're onto a winner!

Cognitive Reframing

This moves us splendidly onto *cognitive reframing*. Cognitive reframing is when we take an original belief and we alter it in a way that means we still believe it but it's from a more positive perspective. For example, "I hate that I'm going to have a panic attack at work." This could be reframed in a way that it becomes more positive, such as "work will be another chance for me to practise being anxious." Here are some examples of cognitive reframing below and we encourage you to make your own:

Original Thought	Cognitive Reframe
"I'm sick of overthinking everything, it doesn't get me anywhere."	"I have a highly intelligent, analytical brain that sometimes gets stuck in anxious loops."
"Last time I went to the mall, my anxiety didn't go away!"	"I was brave enough to go to the mall and do everything despite feeling anxious."
"I'm always making myself anxious."	'At the moment, my anxious response seems to have my attention."
"What if I get scared at the party and need to leave?"	"The party is the perfect opportunity to practise tolerating my anxiety."
"I'm losing my mind and losing control!"	"I feel vulnerable and can notice that I am having the thoughts 'what if I lose control, or lose my mind?'"
"I'm a burden on people at the moment."	'Everyone goes through tough times in their life, this is mine."

Cognitive Reframing is especially important when we look at the importance of exposure, but more specifically, *wilful tolerance*. This is when we are willing to go and feel anxious in any situation, with the knowledge of *why* we are doing it.

Wilful Tolerance

There are many people trying to battle anxiety and who are bravely putting themselves through situations that make them scared, only for them to be scared the next time they approach the situation. For example, someone who is scared to go too far from their home may attempt to do it, but then feel the relief of being back home again. They successfully *tolerated* the trip out, but perhaps it was missing the main ingredient to recovery – that of doing it willingly.

When we approach scary situations willingly, this primes the brain for active rewiring, both of the anxious response for future situations and also our default behaviours and habits surrounding anxious triggers. This means we have to approach situations knowing that it's ok to be scared, because we know we aren't in any real danger and all we are experiencing is a very noticeable discomfort. This means we must abandon thoughts such as "Oh I hope I don't get anxious later" with thoughts such as "ok the next time I get anxious is the perfect time for me to practise tolerating my anxiety in order to tell my brain this is safe."

It's really important to remind ourselves that the brain actually *wants* to turn off the anxious response and is willing to. However, it will only do it when we *show* it that there is no danger. It's a bit like saying *"hey anxious brain with your scary sensations and what if's. I know you want me to avoid and you're going to give me scary scenarios and bodily sensations to convince me to avoid, but I'm just going to do it anyway. Watch me!"*

Try not to "white-knuckle" your way through situations, as this is the opposite to wilful tolerance. Examples of white-knuckling include:

- Checking the clock and counting down until you can 'escape'

- Frantically trying to distract yourself and batting away the thoughts

- Getting drunk in order to get through a situation

- Researching all the escapes beforehand, or during the event

- Relying on another person to get you through the situation

- Overly relying on emotional crutches, such as a mobile phone

White-knuckling behaviours tell the amygdala that the situation is not safe, or is only safe if we constantly monitor and stay hypervigilant. This only reinforces the idea that the anxious brain needs to remain hypervigilant in situations that scare us.

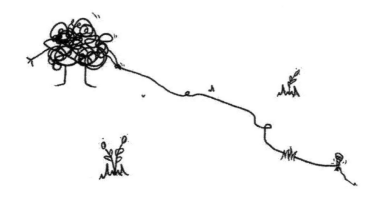

@aprilhillwriting

You must *not* forget that we *practise* this with the attitude of self-compassion. The reason why we use the word *practise* is that we do not expect you to get this absolutely perfect immediately. After any situation when you are anxious, we implore you to pick out the positives of how you did and build upon that – there is no use magnifying and amplifying the negatives.

Inner Dialogue learned from our youth

A lot of how we see anxiety is influenced by beliefs that we learn as a child.

For example, if I am a child crying at a funeral because my grandma passed away, and I turn to my uncle for support but he responds with, "Don't cry! Be strong for your grandma" then imagine what a child might interpret this to mean. What a child might come to understand and *believe* is that they shouldn't cry; that crying is bad or wrong. Perhaps this child is vulnerable around their parents but is met with criticism and disregard. This might lead them to think that it's not ok to be upset. They might *believe* that it's not acceptable to have or express emotions. This contributes to an inner dialogue.

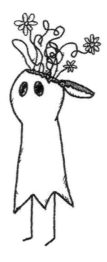

@aprilhillwriting

We learn this inner dialogue during our youth. We derive meaning from the words and behaviours of the people around us which develop into absorbing beliefs about ourselves. Let's take a look at a few examples...

If a child walks up to their dad and tells him that they're upset but the father replies with a sharp, "pull yourself together" then it might have them believing that they are weak. Perhaps this child goes to their mother and explains to her that they are anxious but she turns around and says, "You're anxious? What about me, what about how I feel?" This child might come to believe that it is not ok to be anxious; that other people's feelings are more important than their own.

Similarly, these influences on the inner dialogue can be found in experiences like being bullied at school. Imagine what impact bullying might have on a child. They might absorb the belief that they aren't good enough, that they are pathetic and unworthy of respect.

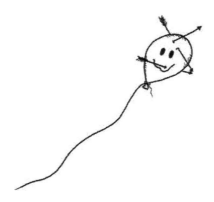

@aprilhillwriting

These beliefs can derive from action or inaction, words said and words that are not said. It is all about what we *infer* from them. The *absence* of hearing "I love you" might encourage a child to absorb a similar belief as if they were told "We never wanted you". They might infer from either scenario that they are not loved and are not worthy of love. Another example might be if a child comes home from school and the parents do not ask how they are. They might *infer* and *interpret* that to mean, "I'm not interesting enough to take notice of".

It is good to reflect on our inner dialogue and how it applies to us now. A lot of people say, "That happened years ago". But, we live by the beliefs that are formulated at that age; the age when our brains are formed. This is why it is beneficial to discuss our inner dialogue using talking therapy. To try and understand where we have learned to talk to ourselves in this way. We can ask ourselves questions like:

· What am I absorbing?

· What am I absorbing about anxiety?

· Do I hold any prejudices?

· Am I prejudiced towards anxiety?

· Do I think it makes me weak?

· Am I ashamed of my anxiety?

When you're feeling anxious and criticising yourself about these feelings it is worth asking, where have I learned this from? Is this the attitude that I want to apply to my recovery from anxiety?

Everyone experiences anxiety in their own way and no one is immune to it; some people just get very good at hiding it. Anxiety is not weakness and it is certainly not something to be ashamed of. Learning to be compassionate with yourself is essential for a lasting recovery.

In Conversation

Josh: Dean how important was it for you to be nice to yourself when you were recovering?

Dean: It was super important because we've got this inner critic haven't we that we've built up since we were a kid, since we were told that we weren't going to be the superhero we thought we would be when we grew up. This inner critic that's always giving you the what-ifs that's always telling you that you're not going to come out of an anxious response- this voice is part of us. So, having to change that narrative was probably one of the most uncomfortable things to do because it requires you going against the inner critic, doesn't it? We must remember that the mind listens and the body reacts. So, if we think something negative the mind will continue to fuel that and then the body will react in a negative way. And when I really sat with that little statement and realized how powerful it was, I started to change the language that I would use and to change that inner narrative.

Josh: It's so important isn't it? I remember what really helped me was quantifying anxiety from one to ten. So, when I was practicing exposure, or just generally kind of measuring my anxiety, I used to think about it like, "Oh it's either on or it's off. I'm either anxious or I'm not." Actually, now it's like, "I'm here at this place and my anxiety is at a four but two weeks ago it was an eight." So, actually I'm going in the right direction, and that's being kind. You're not getting frustrated because you can't just get there immediately, because I think that's one of the biggest stumbling blocks. And that's why we've included cognitive reframing in this book, because it's such a powerful tool to frame things in a positive way.

Dean: And I think Josh it's worth noting that a lot of people when they start to either do your self-help, or therapy, or whatever road they take on recovery, initially they'll get a positive response won't they, but then like any anxiety recovery that isn't a straight line. They'll have setbacks and relapses and it's at that point where you really have to be kind to yourself. You really have to reinforce that you're not in the same position as you were at the start of the anxiety disorder. You've got the psychoeducation now, you know what the anxious response is and you've seen a positive response to this, so that should help you and make you feel more positive going forward.

Josh: Absolutely.

Chapter 8

How to deal with Anxiety Attacks

Featured artist: *@henribipolar*

When discussing the writing of this book, we talked about some really cool ways to deal with anxiety attacks and we'll share them with you in this part of the book.

An anxiety or panic "attack" is when we are flooded with adrenaline in response to stress or an external stressor. Importantly, nothing is actually attacking us, but for some reason the hyperbolic name has been given because lots of adrenaline can feel uncomfortable and overwhelming. The difference between your usual anxiety and experiencing an anxiety attack is when we experience a rush of fear-induced adrenaline, but it catches us off guard and we get *confused*, then we *misinterpret* this as something bigger than it is. An anxiety attack occurs because of the confusion and misinterpretation that can occur around the unexpected dump of harmless adrenaline.

A lot of people then start to feel like they are losing control in some way, because the fear response becomes intense and seems overwhelming. Fear not though, you cannot lose control just because of adrenaline! The mind then starts to race faster than we can keep up with, flooding our minds with lots of *What if?* thoughts that almost seem immediately replaced, one with another:

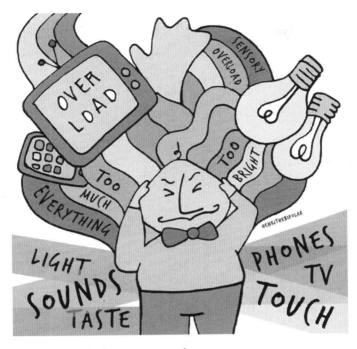

- What if I lose my mind?

- What if I am having a heart attack?

- What if I lose control?

- What if this is something more than anxiety?

- What if this is an undiagnosed physical or psychiatric problem?

Then, to make things even more uncomfortable, we then experience the physical sensations that all the adrenaline and cortisol seem to create. There are many physical symptoms associated with anxiety attacks, but the most common are:

- A state of derealisation/unreality

- Pounding and/or rapid heartbeat

- Struggling to catch breath

- Nausea

- Dizzy or lightheaded

- Muscle tension particularly in chest, jaw and shoulders

- Sweating and hot flushes

So actually anxiety attacks are a mixture of 3 different components: your *emotions*, your *thoughts* and your *sensations*. Interestingly, each anxiety attack can present in different ways; sometimes your heart rate will be rapid, sometimes you won't experience derealisation and other times you may feel flushed and nauseous, but experience nothing else. What is always present during an anxiety attack, though, is *fear*.

Adrenaline rush, not a panic attack

We spoke about cognitive reframing earlier, but one of the best reframes we advise is to change the term "panic attack" or "anxiety attack" to "adrenaline rush" or "adrenaline flood". Not only does this sound less scary, but it is actually more accurate. Remember, the 3 components of an anxiety attack are primarily down to adrenaline; this includes the racing thoughts, the strange sensations and that overarching feeling of fear and doom.

"Hey are you ok?"

"Yeah I'm fine but just experiencing the discomfort of an adrenaline rush at the moment. My mind is racing, my heart is beating fast, my stomach isn't 100% and I feel quite vulnerable, but it is just adrenaline and it will pass soon. Let's carry on."

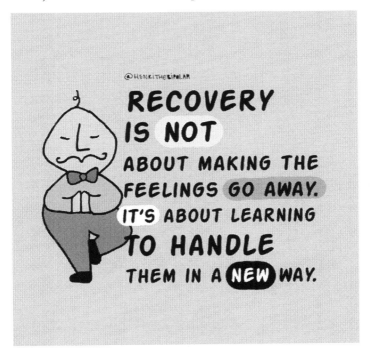

Neuroception

Psychoeducation is so important when it comes to empowering ourselves and building confidence to practise wilful tolerance of anxiety. A really useful part of the anxious response to learn about is the involuntary nervous system and how it relates to us experiencing anxiety.

The involuntary nervous system is the part of our nervous system that runs through our body and is connected to all of our vital organs. It keeps our body running in the background and is responsible for our breathing, our heartbeat, our blood pressure regulation, blood sugar, etc. A lot of anxious people share with us that they often get frightened when their breathing becomes laboured and they can't quite catch their breath. However, we reassure them that they're not actually in charge of their breath and they couldn't stop breathing if they tried. Ultimately, the involuntary nervous system is in charge of keeping our bodies in balance and it does a remarkable job of doing so.

Here's where the involuntary system plays a huge part with anxiety. In order to understand this better, we learn about the two major components: the *sympathetic nervous system* and the *parasympathetic nervous system.*

The Sympathetic Nervous System

The sympathetic nervous system is the part of our nervous system responsible for engaging our *fight, flight or freeze* response. This is the part of our nervous system that can be dictated by the amygdala and is responsible for activating fear and adrenaline. It is also responsible for keeping us 'on edge', by being involved in the process of releasing cortisol to keep us hypervigilant and 'on alert' for dangers. When we are stressed, we engage the sympathetic nervous system to get us through a stressful event, whether this be stress at work, a break up, grief, or social worries, to name a few. This is ok, but – basically put - too much stress, or too much sympathetic activation, can confuse the brain into thinking we are in danger. The amygdala cannot distinguish between an actual threat and the 'threat' caused by stress, so adds more adrenaline just in case we are in danger. This is how a lot of anxiety disorders start.

The Parasympathetic Nervous System

This is the other part of our involuntary nervous system and is responsible for rest, relaxation and digestion. The parasympathetic nervous system is activated when we are resting, socialising, being mindful, distracted by something engaging, sleeping and laughing. It's basically the "fun" part of our nervous system, although to a lot of people, the adrenaline rushes can be fun, too.

The key here is to remember that our involuntary nervous systems need *balance*. Also, when it comes to anxiety attacks, it is helpful to acknowledge that they occur because our sympathetic nervous systems have been overworked and are tired. When this occurs, the sympathetic system becomes hypersensitive, ready to release adrenaline dumps at the slightest sign of danger, distress or shock. Everyone with an anxiety condition has a hypersensitive nervous system.

However, during an anxiety attack, don't put too much emphasis on trying to 'relax' through it. This is almost impossible. The reason why we feel it is helpful to know about the nervous system is to demystify any mystery around *why* we are experiencing a panic attack.

"Oh wow I'm feeling an adrenaline rush. I must have been stressed recently and I know I still have a little bit of lingering fear of anxiety. This is ok, this is just adrenaline and all these feelings and sensations will pass. When they do, I'll make sure to engage my parasympathetic nervous system in order to bring balance back to my body."

Stop trying to resist and fix

When you feel the onset of an anxiety attack, the biggest mistake we can make is to start resisting it or putting up a fight. By resisting, we mean doing our utmost to shut it out, frantically distract, self-medicate or seek immediate reassurances. Unfortunately, when we do this, it suggests to the amygdala that the anxious response itself is something to be feared and fought against. The amygdala gets confused and thinks we need help against a threat, so releases *more* of the adrenaline and cortisol that we are trying to avoid!

The first thing to do is simply acknowledge that this is a threat response. My sympathetic nervous system is stressed, and my amygdala has just released some adrenaline just in case I'm not ok. Of course, we know that anxiety attacks can't hurt us, but the amygdala doesn't care and will provide that extra fuel and energy just in case. As we stated before, this always passes. Adrenaline always passes.

It makes no sense to resist and fight these sensations caused by adrenaline. They will pass on their own and they cannot hurt you. The rapid "what if?" thoughts are just your anxious mind suggesting to you potential reasons why you might be afraid. Just remember the 3 components of anxiety are natural, safe and cannot harm you. Importantly, there is also nothing to "fix" or "work out". Obviously, seeking help for anxiety and talking things through are always beneficial, but trying to work out an anxiety attack just feeds the cycle more. It tells the amygdala that "wow this is a problem and needs to be worked out because it's broken." Unfortunately, the amygdala also interprets this as danger.

Ultimately, when you are anxious, don't you dare stop what you were originally doing. If you stop, change your behaviour, avoid and withdraw because of it, then we are just going to re-enact the same cycle of worry. Instead, reframe an anxiety attack as a time to 'practise' with the anxiety and practise wilful tolerance. If you get hit by an adrenaline dump, the most weird and wonderful suggestion we give to you is you don't have to do anything! Josh's magic rule he wants on a placard in his office is *"do what non-anxious you would do."*

By not reacting, by continuing to do what we were originally doing *despite* the components of anxiety making us feel scared, uncomfortable and doubtful, we are sending an extremely strong message to the amygdala (the conductor of the response) that:

"I would like you to turn this response off as soon as I can and also in the future. It isn't needed now and I'll show you it isn't needed. I no longer fear this response and can show my brain I can continue to live life even with it there. This is just adrenaline. I've got this. This is just adrenaline."

There are a few other tips and tricks in the next section, but in general, the main message is that you don't really have to do anything! Less doing, more being! We both recovered from anxiety because we built up enough knowledge and confidence to be able *not* to react to the anxiety when it arose. The more and more we did this, the better our confidence became and the more we convinced the amygdala to stop releasing copious amounts of adrenaline in response to a trigger. We will share some of our personal tips in the next chapter.

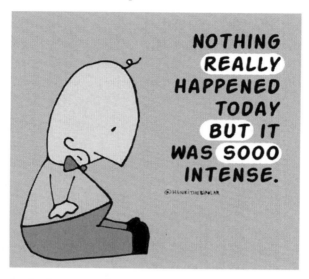

Allow the body to regulate itself

When Josh is sitting in his office opposite a client experiencing an anxiety attack (or 'rush of adrenaline' as we are now going to reframe it), the client might look over to their supportive therapist and receive an unexpected response as Josh simply shrugs his shoulders in plain indifference. To be sure, it's not what they expected but Josh is not cruel, he does this for a very good reason…

Josh: "In my practice, when someone is having an anxiety attack I don't really suggest anything because by reacting to anxiety you're implying that it's dangerous"

This is really important because as we are about to discuss, your body does a magnificent job of bringing you back to a state of equilibrium following a panic attack. Understand that people have a *reactional response* to panic attacks as though the panic attack *itself* is what needs addressing. However, panic attacks occur as a result of prolonged stress, and with this knowledge, we've come to understand that the best thing we can do is *do nothing*. It feels entirely counterintuitive and will go against every feeling in your body that is telling you to respond and 'save yourself' as the nausea in your stomach kicks in and your chest tightens. But here's the thing; when the amygdala sees that you are doing as little as possible, it will realise that panic itself is nothing to be scared of. This is why some people can experience a panic attack and then go back to work while others are so scared of the panic attack that it inhibits their ability to continue on with their day. We forget this. By not reacting to the threat response when we are not in fact in any immediate danger, we are telling it to turn off.

The reason Josh shrugs his shoulders when his clients panic is because neither he nor they need to do anything. Josh is not panicking about his clients, he is calm. Nothing bad is going to happen. And in no less than 20 minutes the clients are often completely fine because together they have shown their threat response that there is no reason to panic. The best thing you can do is not respond to it. Simply do nothing!

It doesn't matter how anxious we get, our bodies have an outstanding ability to always bring us back to a state of balance. The body regulates itself so that you don't have to. When you

117

come out the other side of a panic attack it wasn't because you "used this technique" or you "were lucky" or you "just managed to survive"… It doesn't matter where you are or what you are doing, it is the body that has stabilised you. The body will always find a way to calm you down and bring you back to a harmonious state. Eventually, the adrenaline and cortisol will run out and the nervous systems will intervene, finding stability and bringing you back to normality. **Take this information to be of reassurance because the same control that you are scared of losing is the same lack of control that will bring you back to balance.**

However, it is entirely understandable to want to help yourself in the midst of an anxiety attack. So, if at all possible, you should do your best to do absolutely nothing and show the threat response that it is not needed. But if your anxiety attack is particularly acute and you need to do something to bring yourself into the present, then we have some exercises that might help you.

Understand that these should not be used as tools to 'fix' the problem, merely an aid for tolerating the anxiety attack.

Our first tool is something called a **grounding technique**. This is a very common technique that therapists and trauma therapists use with their clients. A grounding technique can be used in a variety of ways and with this first method we encourage you to stop, take a moment, and try your best to identify five things you can *see*, five things you can *hear*, and five things you can *feel*. Now, you can always hear five different sounds whether that be your heartbeat, the wind, a neighbour, the creaking of a floorboard, cars driving past, someone's music, the birds in the sky, or even a running shower. When we think about identifying things that we can feel these could include things like temperature, clothes on your skin, the chair under your bottom, the socks on your feet, or the rug beneath your bare toes.

Once you've identified five things; move on to four, then move on to three, then two, and finally one.

One of our favourite grounding techniques is to look around, say what we see, and then think of two descriptive adjectives that we could use to describe our chosen object. For example, you might be walking through a park and you say what you see, "I see a tree". With this technique, however, we find those two descriptive adjectives and think instead, "I see an old, oak tree". Another example; "I see a car" becomes "I see a rusty, vintage-looking car". The trick is to focus on the details of the object and describe it in greater depth, this helps to root us firmly in the present. It is worth caveating this technique with something really important – this is really difficult to do. It is not easy and it's not supposed to be! Regardless, you can attempt to *do it anyway*. The reason being that the threat response will register that you're ignoring it and that you're trying to do something in the present. By focusing on staying grounded in the present we can more easily ignore the threat response which will help us to turn it off when it isn't needed.

So, that's two of our favourite grounding techniques.

Let's move on to the seemingly controversial topic of 'the breath'. A lot of yogis around the world will teach you to 'focus on the breath' and while that can be incredibly helpful for many in practising mindfulness etc, for some, concentrating on their breathing during an anxiety attack isn't actually helpful. On the contrary, it could have the opposite effect to the desired one! When faced with a wise old yogi who would calmly reinforce that we should follow their guidance and 'focus on the breath' an anxiety sufferer may well feel the urge to scream at them:

"No! I have a panic disorder, why would I focus on my breath? If I focus on how terrible my breathing is when I'm already aware of how terrible my breathing is, it's only going to make me panic more! So, no, I won't focus on my breath, thank you!"

The truth of the matter is that asking someone to concentrate on their breath in the middle of a panic attack is considered the go-to advice but in all likelihood, it could exacerbate the problem. With that said, if concentrating on your breath doesn't add any secondary fear, then we have a breathing technique that you can try. The technique is very simple; put one hand on your belly and push your belly out with every inhale. This is exactly how we are supposed to breathe. If you notice babies when they sleep, you can see their stomachs rise and fall and this is because their breath goes into their bellies. You can watch as their little round tums go up and down, up and down. However, thanks to social conditioning, we breathe into our chest because it is not considered 'socially acceptable' to walk around with anything other than flat, washboard abs. So, we don't like to breathe how nature intended because that would mean allowing our gut to hang out, and apparently, people don't want to see that.

If you decide to give this belly breathing exercise a go, there is no specific amount of time that you should be breathing for but just make sure that your 'out' breath is one second longer than your 'in' breath. By doing this you are exhaling more carbon dioxide and taking in less oxygen which brings everything back to balance. Belly breathing, over time, will trigger the parasympathetic nervous system (our rest and digest response) which allows us to remain calm and in control. Let's get one thing straight, do not take three deep belly-breaths and check to see if your anxiety is gone, that's not going to work! It's an exercise that can encourage this response over time so once again, this is not a 'fix' but simply a tool to help you tolerate an anxiety attack.

Ultimately it's a case of trusting your body to do its job. The body will always regulate itself. No matter what state of panic you find yourself in, eventually the adrenaline will run out and your body will restore itself to its natural balance. Whilst you can use these coping exercises above, you must trust that your body knows what it's doing. It knows how to handle itself and it knows how to bring things back to a state of equilibrium... even when you feel out of control, your body is fully in control.

In Conversation

Josh: I'm drawing from personal experience here, I remember when I got really confident with panic attacks or anxiety attacks, or as we like to call them, adrenaline rushes, and I used to just say three things to myself. Not as a magic spell to get rid of anxiety, but just as reassurance to myself – "this is just adrenaline and this is just anxiety, it will pass and you can cope." I used to say that to myself, and it was right every time. You know I didn't necessarily feel it every time, oh you know, because anxiety's main purpose is to make you doubt. "Okay my mind's rushing, my heart's pounding. I don't feel here. I feel detached. All right. Well, this must be adrenaline. This must be my anxious response. You know let's go for it!" And then I would basically say to myself, "What would I usually be doing right about now?" then I would go and commit my attention to that instead because I need to teach the amygdala - my anxious brain - there's no imminent danger here and I'm going to show it. The first time I did this, I was so proud, because it's very hard, and then it gets easier and easier and easier.

What advice would you give for an anxiety attack?

Dean: So, just going back to the situation at the office, looking back, I didn't really take any time away from the situation, even in the middle of the panic attack. I did, however, take some time off to help with the grieving of my father. But when I went back into work, I was still in the center of a panic disorder. So, I was waking up and accepting the anxiety and panic every day, I'd wake up put my watch on and then be like "yep, here's nine hours in work, what's anxiety going to bring to me today?" Like you said, labeling anxiety for what it is, is really important; it's really useful. And when I was first in the office what I'd do- I'd always almost create a safety behavior of getting up out of my seat and running. I'll go into the toilet to try and compose myself. Yes, again, initially it would help because I would do like breathing techniques to reduce the anxiety. But what would happen is I'd go back into the office, and I'd get the response again. The reason is because I'm using the safety behavior and avoiding the anxiety. Aren't I? I'm avoiding the situation. So, what I did was sit with the anxiety. I sat with it. We know what it's going to throw at us. We know it's going to be uncomfortable. We know that it's even going to convince us that this time, it's going to be different than last time. But we know from the evidence that every time it does go away. It is temporary. It isn't permanent.

Josh: Brilliant. Yeah, I remember mine, it's not temporary, it's not permanent, and calling it's bluff- just calling its bluff was one. And also, nobody knows, but if you're angry, use this to your advantage and channel the anger towards that anxiety; I did that and it really helped [laughs] you know. But anger gets a lot of bad press you know, "You shouldn't be angry." No, use the anger; use it for exposure and I think it can be really helpful.

But a big one is when someone said to me, "The body will always regulate itself. It's got a fantastic ability to regulate itself and bring you back to balance." And trust it too; it's clever. Your body does not want to maintain this anxiety, so yeah, it's going to regulate itself and that's something that stuck with me to this day.

Dean: That's brilliant and I think it's just worth knowing the difference - you can have a panic attack which sometimes is called an anxiety attack. But there are differences between types of anxiety that people might get during the day, either like a gradual build up, to a full-blown fight or flight or freeze situation where it's a complete adrenaline flood.

Chapter 9

Our Handpicked Tips & Hints

Featured Artist: @missprincesia

Scale your anxiety

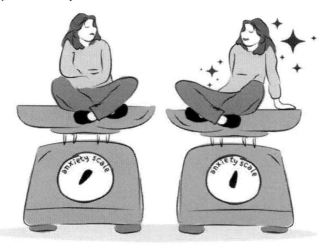

@missprincesia

We can't begin to tell you how helpful it is to scale your anxiety. Scaling your anxiety between a score of 1 to 10 is helpful for many reasons:

- It helps you to see anxiety is something that constantly changes and fluctuates.

- You can see small reductions and increases in anxiety in relation to behaviours and triggers.

- It helps you to *observe* anxiety and expect the symptoms before they occur.

- It's easier to measure progress.

Progress in overcoming anxiety is often measured in steps or stages. By scaling our anxiety, we can challenge any self-doubt or critical thoughts by drawing upon our anxiety in certain situations and using them as factual evidence for progress. For example, "oh my god I'm still anxious when I go to the grocery store." Could be cognitively reframed - with the aid of scaling our anxiety – to "I'm in the grocery score with an anxiety score of 5, instead of the usual 9 or 10. I'm getting better at wilful tolerance."

Another example could be, "I'm at a 6 in the morning when I wake up. I used to be a 9, so I've done something right so far." When practising exposure, scaling can be really helpful because you can notice the numbers start to fall when you have been with the triggering situation long enough. A good exposure session is when you stay with the fear, without "white-knuckling" or relying on reassurance, and you begin to notice that your anxiety levels are coming down. This is a core tenet of recovery.

The next time anxiety suggests to you "what if this lasts forever?" or "what if this is now you forever?" then simply refer to your anxiety scores. "Well actually, anxiety, I was at a 3 yesterday when I was tidying up, so it can't possibly mean this is me forever. This is just adrenaline and I'm working on my fear of you."

Stop monitoring and score points

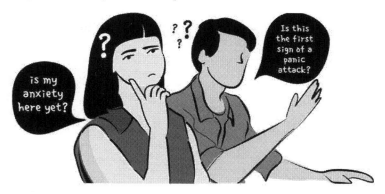

If you've lived with anxiety for a while, you will be very familiar with the compulsion of checking ourselves and scanning our body for the signs of anxiety. We do this because we fear anxiety and the discomfort that it produces. We can also monitor for the first sign of 'disaster' happening that is external to us. Perhaps one or more of these statements will resonate with you:

- "Is my anxiety here yet?"

- "Is this the first sign of a panic attack?"

- "Is this strange symptom something sinister? I'll keep an eye on it."

- "Are they angry at me? I'll monitor just in case."

- "If I keep this worry in mind, I'll be prepared for when it does happen."

- "Surely if I ruminate enough on this problem, then I can find the solution."

These thoughts often turn into actions, or more accurately referred to as 'compulsions'. It is the compulsion to check and the habit that keeps the amygdala on alert. Please remember:

The more we check and monitor ourselves for the anxiety, the longer it wants to stick around. It is impossible to stop checking and monitoring straight away, but less checking means less anxiety.

With less checking and monitoring, comes less anxiety (read in the *Spiderman voice*). With this in mind, Josh devised a game to play, which also factors in cognitive reframing. The game is simple: every time you catch yourself checking on your anxiety, or monitoring and ruminating, count the amount of minutes, hours or seconds you have just spent *not* doing that. Instead of getting frustrated and disciplining yourself for checking, we want you to immediately reframe this into a positive, then give yourself some points:

"Ok I've caught myself checking for signs of illness again. However, I went 4 minutes without doing this. That's 4 points to me!"

This game can be very powerful and is also a good way to literally rewire the brain when it comes to associations with anxious behaviours. It also applies when we have been feeling calm for a long time, then suddenly get caught off guard by an adrenaline dump. Rather than assuming the anxiety is back for good and is ready to plague you until the end of time, here is a chance to say "oh wow, I have been weeks without thinking about how I feel. I feel uncomfortable now, but I need to remind myself of this."

This ties into talking to yourself with kindness and compassion like we mentioned earlier in the book.

How you score the points, record them and reward yourself, is up to you. You can pop them in a journal, an app on your phone, vocally with someone else or just mentally store them as a rough guide. When you reach a certain total of points, promise yourself a treat, such as an evening off or buying yourself something nice!

Engage the present

Have you ever walked past a school playground and noticed most kids are running around, having fun and, importantly, are engaged in the present? You don't see them sitting in the corner, deeply lost in thought, about their anxiety disorders and trying to fix themselves. Obviously, there are some children who do struggle emotionally, but in general, when you walk past a school playground, it is a vibrant, energetic place emanating laughter, playful screams and optimistic energy.

Anxiety disorders convince you that it is not ok to stay in the present moment. Think about it, every "what if?" is based in the future, or when we are dwelling on something in the past. These "what if?"s are usually scary in nature, then when you couple them with uncomfortable sensations and emotions, they suddenly have all of your attention. In contrast, every person who isn't anxious will spend a lot of their day with thoughts and attention in the present. What this looks like is different for each individual.

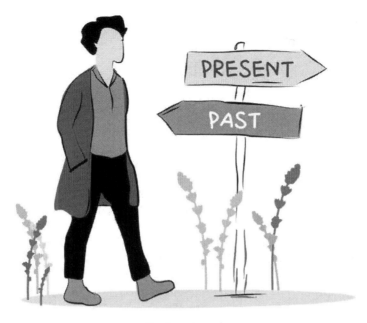

@missprincesia

"Non-anxious me would just walk around daydreaming and playing with my imagination about cool stuff. I'd also just be enjoying stuff in front of me. This was me being in my present – not engaging with the very persuasive scary thoughts and sensations that my threat response was trying to signal." - Josh

Interestingly, focussing on the present is the central tenet of *mindfulness*. Mindfulness is a branch of meditation with the sole intention of bringing us into the present. It is often suggested as a panacea for mental health conditions (which it isn't) but it is a very useful practise to get involved with as it helps us with our aim of keeping our thoughts and attention in the present.

When our thoughts are in the present, the mind and body return to a state of balance quicker than when we try to rush it. Think about it, if you have ever been busy, or distracted, then you would have probably noticed that the anxiety is less than when it has our whole attention. Unfortunately, people misuse mindfulness as a 'technique' to eradicate anxiety, which often does not work, particularly for people struggling with a fear of fear. "I've tried mindfulness and it didn't work!"

We recommend using mindfulness as a pre-emptive measure when you're calmer. This will help us prepare to use it for when we are anxious and when we are practising wilful tolerance. If you wait until you are panicking to try and use mindfulness, you'll realise it's very difficult to focus on anything else but a frantically fast mind.

In summary, start practising being in the present, whether it's through the discipline of mindfulness, or just practising engaging with things in your life that are in front of you. This will be different for each individual. We're back to Josh's golden rule again: *"do what non anxious you would do and commit to it."* Furthermore, when combined with our point scoring game of counting the times we are not monitoring and checking, keeping our focus on things in the present is a real winner.

Less doing, more being. The body fixes itself.

If anxiety and panic cannot hurt us, then rationally, why would we need to do something about it if it arose? Why would we need to fix or correct anything? One of the biggest mistakes is thinking we need to do something when we are anxious. If you are a person who does this, consider if anything that you have 'done' has worked yet? We suggest actually doing nothing. This outrageously means practising doing nothing and seeing what happens. No rushing to Dr Google, or asking for reassurance, or rushing for supplements, or running to a safe space. Do nothing.

There's method to our madness, because of the role of the amygdala. If the amygdala is signalling danger and sounding the alarm, it expects us to act, either via fight or flight. What do you think we are showing the amygdala when we choose to do neither of these? How do you think the amygdala responds when we haven't really changed what we are doing for a while? Anxious recovery is more about *being*, than *doing*. This comes with practise.

The Alarm Analogy

A good tip we like to share with people we work with is to draw upon the metaphor of a *false alarm*. Imagine you are sat at home and your fire alarm starts sounding. What do you do? Well hopefully you would be startled into action; you would quickly check to see if there was fire, perhaps smell for smoke and shout to loved ones, then get the hell out of there and wait for the fire brigade. You may even be able to extinguish the source of a small fire yourself, for instance if you realised that you had left the oven on, or if your hairdryer overheats. This is the whole function of the fire alarm, to warn you that there could be potential danger. The alarm triggers and sounds the same whether there is a whiff of smoke, or if the building is burning down.

The amygdala uses adrenaline and cortisol to set off the body's alarm system and we invite you to conceptualise your anxious/threat response like this. This alarm system, when highly stressed, can go off at any 'whiff' of danger or stress. However, like any alarm at home, there most likely isn't a fire, but it triggers 'just in case' there is one. Importantly, if our fire alarm goes off at home, we most likely do not behave like there is a fire initially, but we may check out of intrigue anyway. People with an anxiety disorder, however, react to their own alarm system as if there is a fire every time it sounds.

Imagine you are in an office building doing some work when the building safety officer visits and announces that he will be testing the fire alarm within the next hour. He claims you are not required to do anything as it is just a test to see if it is working. He visits every month and it's no big deal. So you continue with your emails and begin writing quite a detailed paragraph, when suddenly you are startled by the sound of a loud, screeching siren. The sound makes you jump, and for a brief second you feel like you are in danger. Then, at that moment, you recall that this is a fire alarm test – this is a false alarm – and you remind yourself that you do not need to do anything. Despite the loud siren, you are able to continue with your emails, with the siren in the background. After all, you're used to this by now.

This is exactly how we should perceive anxiety and adrenal rushes. People who react to false alarms in their body will immediately drop what they are doing and be called into action. They stop doing their emails and run outside just in case there is fire – even though they have been foretold that there will be a false alarm. This is what people who fear and misinterpret anxiety do. Every time they get an alarm, via the amygdala signalling the activation of fight or flight, they immediately assume it is real and that imminent peril is around the corner. Following on from the last section, let's practise not reacting to false alarms!

Parasympathetic activities

Instead of relying on reacting to anxiety when it arises, why don't we work on preventative measures in our day-to-day lives? As mentioned in the *Anxiety Attacks* chapter, we really believe in working on the balance of our involuntary nervous system. Anxious people have an overstimulated sympathetic nervous system, so we must work on bringing balance (to the force?) by engaging our *parasympathetic* nervous system.

This includes an effort to factor emotionally nourishing activities into our lives. This includes:

- Having fun – giving yourself permission to enjoy something for you and also as a means to combat anxiety.

- Meditation – can work wonders but isn't for everyone.

- Deep breathing practice.

- Laughing – having a laugh either on your own (watching a comedy or something) or laughing with friends and family is excellent for this.

- Running a hot bath.

- Getting a massage.

- Mild exercise (nothing too exhaustive).

- Being within nature.

- Eating wholesome and delicious food.

- Relaxation – this includes just taking a break and lying down, perhaps with a book or tv.

- Gaming – playing video games that are not intense and stressful. Try to avoid first-person shooters and horror games.

- Yoga and Tai Chi.

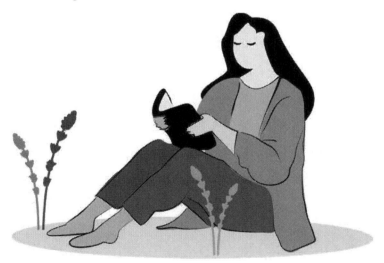

@missprincesia

It is important to make sure you find out what works for you and to not fall into the trap of doing what you "should" be doing. Don't try to replicate other people if it is not working for you. Personally we don't practise much yoga, but we know it helps many people we know.

Making something else the centre of your life

When we've had anxiety for so long it can become the centre of our lives.

Every day we wake up trying to fix it. We try to find the solution, the answer. We imagine that if we just dig deep, go inwards and explore the different layers within inception, that maybe we can find the solution. Each and every day we are searching for answers because with every sunrise we open our eyes and can immediately feel the weight of our anxiety. It can fully consume us until everything we do revolves around managing our worries. The idea that we can think our way out of it, keep searching and ruminating until we somehow find an answer is a sure-fire path to remaining in this anxious cycle.

This only subscribes to a romanticised view that anxiety is something you can fix inside your head. With a good therapist you can explore and conceptualise your anxiety but you, on your own, going around and around in thought loops, isn't going to achieve anything.

Of course, if we've been anxious for a long time, we might not know what a non-anxious life looks like anymore. It becomes an unhelpful mental habit and, like all unhelpful habits, they are notoriously tough to break. This is why there are tools and techniques to help you and the one we are going to discuss here is all about making something else the centre of your life. How do you do that? You have to plan it out. You must ask yourself what you would be doing if you weren't anxious? What exactly does a non-anxious week look like?

Josh has been working through this technique with a client in his practice and helping them outline a weekly schedule. Let's compare an anxious day to a non-anxious day:

On an anxious day, this person might wake, open their eyes and think about how they feel. Immediately they worry. This feeling of worry means that they can't eat breakfast because they now feel nauseous or find themselves too distracted with concern. So, they do what we all do and look to Google for advice and reassurance. Perhaps they read through some books to help find some answers or flick through their social media for guidance, for stories they can relate to. They try to keep themselves busy in a bid to avoid their anxiety, maybe they do some cooking or cleaning, but at the end of the day, they are exhausted. All of the adrenaline and worry has drained them of their energy and they go to bed feeling fatigued and stressed.

Now, assuming everything else remains the same, what might they do if they weren't anxious? Our client here might be inclined to say, "Well, I'd likely wake up and go to eat breakfast. But if I'm too anxious, I won't be able to eat it." The answer here is to do it anyway. With each task in our day to day lives that might be interrupted or hindered by the presence of anxiety, we must do them anyway because that is what you want to train the brain to do. If you can only take two bites of that breakfast then great!

Who cares?! You've done it. You're already doing something different from what you were before. You are already taking the steps to turn off that threat response.

Plan out what a normal week looks like for you and commit to it.

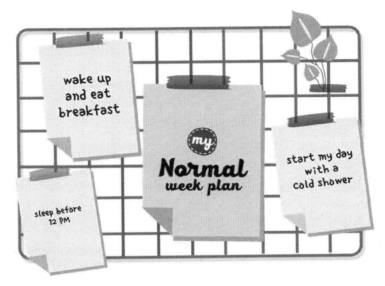

@missprincesia

The reason this technique is so great is because it rewires the brain. Anxiety thrives in habit, so you can think about how every day is Groundhog Day when we live with anxiety at the core of everything we do and every decision we make. We wake up, do the anxious bit and we go to sleep but alas; the anxiety hasn't gone away. We haven't found the answer, we haven't found the solution, we have simply lived another day exactly the same as the day before and the day before that. Something has to change.

Anxiety goes away when you ask it to go away. And, when you repeat it for long enough, the new habit becomes the main habit and the old habit fades away. In the same way that a person might struggle to give up an addiction like smoking, we become addicted to the habit – we become addicted to the search for relief. Let's change that by interrupting the thought loop. And how do we interrupt the thought loop? We plan our days and commit to them as if we were living a non-anxious life.

In Conversation

Josh: For me what I really found useful was to not try and activate the parasympathetic nervous system as a reaction to when I'm *already anxious* or when I'm *already* panicking. Obviously, do it if you're stressed and things, but sometimes when we've been ignoring stress for so long and then suddenly, we find ourselves panicking, that then isn't the time to go and practice meditation, this isn't the time to go and run an ice bath. Because it's arguably too late, so do it after the panic has finished, and for me that was massive. It was preventative rather than reactionary. I just think you know so many people disregard things- helpful things like meditation because of things like, "Oh yeah I tried meditation". Well yeah you tried it when you were panicking as a remedy to calm yourself down - you know you tried it as a reaction, but actually what's really helpful if you meditate when calm, put it as part of your routine.

Dean: I like that Josh. And I think the perfect way of saying that is that people are trying to use this as a *tool* - I probably fell into this category as well when I was first looking at tools to help overcome anxiety. Some people use meditation or mindfulness in the peak of panic and try and use it as a crutch, don't they?

Josh: Yes.

Dean: Whereas, like you say, it's good to implement as a preventative measure. So, the things that helped for me was mindfulness - just being present, so what you said about labeling the anxiety is actually something that arises as a skill from practising mindfulness. So, when I was feeling anxious, I'd be mindful that I was feeling anxious and I knew what it was. Another helpful tool for me was correct breathing. So, I don't know if you know Josh, but over 70% of us breathe incorrectly, so we don't breathe using what it is called belly breathing; we don't breathe through the belly and we take shorter breaths. Like you with meditation, practising this when I was not panicking was helpful, but I know a lot of people can struggle if they try to do it as a reaction to acute panic, rather than practising when we are calm.

Josh: That's a really good one. Another trick that really helped me was scaling; I've mentioned it before, but scaling anxiety and working with other people to communicate my anxiety score. So, rather than constantly repeating myself to my friends, loved ones, my partner, "Oh I'm anxious! I'm anxious." I'd say, "I'm a six." "Oh okay, so you're fairly anxious." "Yeah. Oh, I'm a nine. I'm a nine. Oh, you really must be panicking." "I'm a two." "Oh, brilliant because this morning you were a nine." And I think that's really important.

Dean: Yeah. And that's obviously a really good CBT technique that's tried and tested, isn't it? This scaling of the anxiety response so the clients can see the anxiety scale, it isn't a yes or a no, it isn't an on or an off switch, it is a sliding scale. And like you say, being aware of where you are on this scale, can be really useful and really helpful with loved ones or family members or work colleagues. And just touching on what you said earlier, even when I first started dealing with anxiety and panic, what I would do was just keep it all in my mind, so I'd be in the office, or be out with my friends, and I would just keep it all to myself and almost have this internal battle with myself. And what I found useful was that I turn around to my friend and I would say, "Listen just letting you know I feel a bit anxious at the moment." And they'd say, "Do you know what, ah so do I." And you wouldn't believe it, would you, that the people around you are having their own internal battles? So, that's why I think it is really important that we're all there to help each other, and not be scared of telling people that you're feeling anxious. You can get this from journaling as well; getting thoughts from the mind out onto a piece of paper helps. You're moving it away from the irrational thoughts process in your mind, aren't you?

Josh: Absolutely. I think for me the most important- well one of the most important things is compassion. You must try and be nice to yourself and try and catch yourself being self-critical because no one has ever overcome anxiety from being extremely self-critical. You cannot criticize yourself out of an anxiety disorder; and that has to be remembered. Talk to yourself like you talk to a loved one, or to a good friend and that's the way you can encourage yourself out of it; I think that's really important.

Dean: Yes. When you initially get clients coming to you, or you might have been asked on your Instagram platform, but do you get frequently asked questions like, "How do I get rid of anxiety?" "How do I get rid of overthinking?" "How do I stop irrational thoughts?"

So, I think highlighting the psychoeducation around that it's not the thought, it's your reaction to it and your behavior in response to the thoughts that is really important.

Chapter 10

Success Stories from the Community

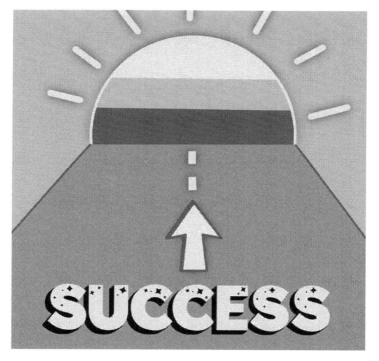

We thought it would be helpful to include some recounts from members of our community that talk about their successes. The section includes a selection of stories sent in by members. We have anonymised people's names by changing them:

Sally's story with Panic Disorder

Hey guys, it all started one day when I suddenly felt a bit weird when I was at work. By 'weird', I mean I felt spaced-out and it was like I was questioning my reality all of a sudden. I now know this is called derealisation. Anyway, my initial thought was suddenly "oh my god, what if I am losing my mind?". To add to this, I suddenly started panicking over what was happening, my heart started to race and I began to sweat. More rapid "what if?" thoughts started to flood my mind, such as "what if you're having a heart attack?", which just added to my overall panic.

I looked around desperately looking to my colleagues for help, but their faces looked far away and the looks of concern on their faces only added to my worry. I pleaded for someone to call an ambulance, which they did. The paramedics arrived and gave me the once over and took me to the hospital as a precaution. I had several tests, including an ECG of my heart, and they all came back fine. Initially I was relieved, but a few days later the fear and the strange, 'spaced out' feeling returned again.

I took time off work and stayed at home, thinking it was a good idea to stay indoors and try to 'work out' how I felt. I paced my room, ruminating and analysing why I suddenly felt the way I did. I kept waking up with this sense of dread and doom that would not shift. My feelings had all my attention and days went by with no progress. How I felt affected my sleep, eating and digestion, which yet again added yet more worry to the worry pile.

It was only after discovering you guys that I began to realise that there wasn't actually anything wrong with me. You also signposted me to relevant resources that my doctor and the hospital failed to do. To be honest, I'd never really resonated with the word 'anxiety', I just thought it was a word that worriers used to describe their feelings about everyday worries. Yet there I was, feeling anxious!

What helped me to recover was knowing that monitoring and focussing on harmless effects of anxiety and adrenaline was keeping me in the anxious cycle. Also, it really helped to see that my anxiety problem was more of a *phobia,* than an illness. I had developed a phobia of the symptoms of anxiety; I was terrified of panicking! Obviously, this was difficult to observe when I initially had my first panic attack, as I had no idea what was happening. Now I know it was my fight-or-flight activating because of prolonged stress.

Knowing that anxiety couldn't hurt me and that it was a natural bodily response helped me to change my attitude and behaviour towards the panic. I stopped avoiding and actually practised being anxious in situations where I was initially doubtful of challenging.

My aim was clear, I wanted to eradicate the *secondary fear* that you speak about – the worry about worry and I did this by identifying all of my safety and avoidance behaviours, such as staying at home, pacing my room and trying to 'solve' the problem mentally. To do this, I practised wilful tolerance of anxiety and panic. Soon enough, I realised panic attacks are just adrenaline rushes that cause strange symptoms that go alongside them. I was willing to let my heart rate increase, I was willing to feel derealised and spaced out, I just let my breath become laboured. Lo and behold, the anxiety passes, because the adrenaline runs out. The body stops releasing cortisol also, which then made me stop feeling 'on-edge'.

I grew in confidence and slowly got my life back. I even looked forward to challenging myself as I realised anxiety is just discomfort, not danger. I hope this helps someone. If you have been in a similar situation to me, then you can do it!

Sally.

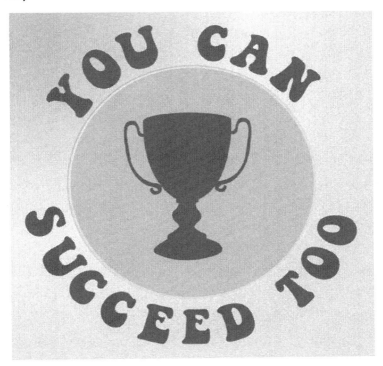

Faisal's story with Agoraphobia

Hey guys, thank you so much for what you do, especially for helping me over the last few months. I'd be more than happy to summarise my story for you.

My agoraphobia started a few years back when I slowly started to restrict the things that I would do in my life. I now know it first started when I refused to go on holiday abroad, because I had an anxiety attack when I was in Spain one time. My vacations from then on were localised in the UK but I didn't properly acknowledge what was happening. I also started to avoid driving on motorways and busy roads, choosing to take the longer, quieter routes instead. When I really noticed there was a problem, however, was when I was out walking in the hills with my wife and I experienced a 'panic attack', or what I now know as a rush of adrenaline. This frightened me so much that I immediately turned back and went home. Of course, this is when I stopped going for walks, which I usually love doing.

I asked work if I could work from home for a while, which they allowed and I spun some excuses as to why. I set up my office in the spare room and got into the habit of working from home. As time went by, I realised I didn't need to leave the house. My wife did the shopping and, when it was my turn, I ordered the shopping to be delivered. This façade didn't last for long though and my wife began to question me because she was concerned.

My agoraphobia kept me inside by suggesting thoughts and scenarios in my mind about me 'freaking out' if I attempted to leave the house. I had made my house my 'safe zone', but in reality it didn't help me staying inside. Looking back, I realise that my safe zone had been changing over time, by shrinking and shrinking since the moment I experienced anxiety whilst in Spain. It shrank even more when I started to restrict myself to certain routes to work, then finally confining myself to my home. My anxiety had successfully managed to get me to avoid the outside using scary thoughts and sensations. Ultimately, I stayed home "just in case" something awful happened if I left the house. However, if I really peel it back, I didn't leave the house because I was afraid of how it would make me *feel*. Agoraphobia is a fear of fear, where the mind just suggests nonsense to you in order to get you to avoid.

To recover, I reversed all of this. I practised wilful tolerance and tried to do things without "white-knuckling" my way through them. I also spoke to a counsellor and my wife about how harsh on myself I could be and this helped me to apply a more accepting attitude when it came to a successful, but patient, recovery. I also educated myself on what was happening in my body and learned invaluable insights from DLCAnxiety and AnxietyJosh. I constantly reminded myself that "this is just anxiety" and that it cannot hurt me.

It also helped to understand why my home became the safe place and why I hardly ever experienced anxiety there. This is because, every time I experienced an anxious episode, I would withdraw to my home. Importantly, every time my anxiety subsided, I always seemed to be in my house – my amygdala was registering an unhelpful message that the only place I was seeming to calm down was in my house. With this knowledge, it made so much sense as to why I was more and more reluctant to go anywhere else!

I knew I had recovered when I went on a long walk with my wonderful wife and I started to experience shortness of breath and feeling a horrible sense of doom. I felt the urge to run, but I didn't. Not so long afterwards, the anxiety subsided. I slowed down a little, but I didn't stop walking. Knowing that anxiety can and will pass wherever I am was the most empowering fact to learn when overcoming anxiety. A big thanks to you guys for educating me on this.

Best, Faisal.

Monique's story with Generalised Anxiety

I had always been a worrier since I was a child, but ever since becoming a mum my anxiety went off the charts! I couldn't get through 10 minutes without worrying about something. What really helped me was understanding the process and function behind worry. My worry was a by-product of my *threat response* that was trying to look after me. My threat response – trying to keep me safe – was constantly monitoring my life for threats and suggesting catastrophes to me. For so long I engaged with these thoughts because I thought that, if I worry about something, I can prevent the disaster from happening. This just kept me worrying all the time, though. Since having kids, I realised I didn't have all the resources to maintain this unhelpful worry cycle.

Over time, and thanks to learning about anxiety and GAD, I realised that it was *safe* not to engage with the constant "what if?"s my brain was throwing at me. What was more difficult though, was practising not engaging with the feeling of uncertainty and danger that GAD always throws at you. I got really good at disengaging from the worry and committing my attention elsewhere to the present. I got really good at observing my patterns of behaviour and worry and rewarded myself when I caught myself ruminating. Anxiety can be such a sly devil!

For me, overcoming GAD was about turning off my threat response by showing the anxious mind that I was not in any danger. I also reframed how I saw GAD – I now see it as a protective system of my body that wants to keep me safe, but it is willing to turn off if I let it. Nowadays I am doing well. Sometimes thoughts become sticky, but I remind myself that where my focus is is what is important. If I keep focusing on scary thoughts and sensations, then they continue. A big hurdle is giving yourself permission to guide your focus away (although I know it feels unsafe!)

If you have GAD, you are not broken, there is nothing wrong with you, but there are a few things you can tweak to make your life better.

Gavin's story with Health Anxiety

Hey Dean and Josh,

As you know my story with health anxiety lasted for years because I didn't have the right knowledge and help. To put it simply, every time I noticed or felt something unusual, it would trigger my anxious response and I would get sucked into the really scary scenarios that my anxious brain was suggesting to me. If my heart skipped a beat, I'd assume it was a heart defect, or "what if this is a heart defect?". If I had a headache, I'd assume it was a brain tumour. If I had an unusual symptom, I'd commit the absolute anxious atrocity of googling the symptom, only to end up even more frightened than I initially was! Health anxiety consumed my life.

Now I know that my amygdala triggered my anxiety in response to unusual triggers and made me *doubt* that I was safe. I am now aware that the anxious response made me doubt that random symptoms were harmless because that is the whole purpose of anxiety. Anxiety is supposed to make me doubt so it has my attention and that I stay on alert for potential 'dangers'. Instead of stepping back and acknowledging this, I engaged with the scary thoughts and sensations as if each trigger was real, which just kept me in a habit of assuming every symptom was a sign of my imminent demise.

I'd seek reassurance from people around me. I'd constantly ring my doctor, ask for advice on social media groups and forums and trawl the internet for that relief and reassurance that I thought I was desperately in need of. What I didn't realise was that I was making the anxious response and its content the centre of my life when it occurred. When I learned to allow the anxious response to be there, not engage immediately and seek empty reassurance, I noticed that my anxious response started to come down. When the anxious response, or as Josh calls it 'the threat response' calmed down, I started to see things with more clarity again.

The skill with health anxiety is to learn not to immediately engage with it. I knew, deep down, that my symptom was a symptom of anxiety, but resisting the urge to drop everything immediately and give it my full attention was the biggest hurdle. I can safely say that I can do this now. I'm happy because the more I've practised this over the last few months, the less and less the anxiety and sticky thoughts consume me.

Gav

Mairead's story with OCD

Hi Josh and Dean, here is my story of living with OCD.

Growing up I lived with typical OCD behaviours. I couldn't stop washing my hands and I had to tap the doorknob ten times before leaving a room. If I didn't do these things, I had an intense feeling that something bad would happen. If I didn't wash my hands then I would worry that I'd somehow contaminate and kill my family. Likewise, if I didn't tap the doorknob ten times then I'd panic that someone would break into the house and burgle us.

But it went beyond these typical OCD behaviours as I had developed other mental compulsions. At night, if I didn't picture my loved ones' faces in great detail (and in the 'correct' order) then something terrible would happen to them.

However, as I grew up, I noticed that I stopped exhibiting these behaviours for reasons that were unknown to me at the time. Perhaps I was distracted with life but, regardless of the reasons why I was fine and free from OCD up until my twenties. During my twenties, I developed an anxiety disorder after experiencing a panic attack. I was so scared of the panic attack itself and so scared of health anxiety that the OCD habits that I had somehow rid myself of, returned. This time it came back in the form of self-monitoring, checking, and scanning for signs of panic or signs of health anxiety.

I noticed that some of my old OCD behaviours had also re-emerged; I found myself cleaning excessively, far too often. This was not helped by the involvement of the pandemic, as you can imagine. I was aware of the reappearance of compulsive cleaning but luckily, being mostly at home during this time, that particular behaviour didn't affect me too much. But, what was really unhelpful was the obsessive monitoring and self-scanning which kept triggering my threat response.

I found myself caught in an endless loop of triggering the threat response, which triggered the compulsive checking and monitoring, which further triggered the threat response! By constantly searching for a reason behind the panic and trying to end the cycle, I was in fact encouraging it to continue. This became quite debilitating for me.

By learning about anxiety and how the threat response works from you, Josh and Dean, I realized that OCD is about turning off that threat response. It suddenly all made sense. I realized that I overcame my first bout of OCD when I took my attention *away* from the threat response. Ultimately, my OCD left when I got my first job where I was busy and distracted. Because I guided my attention away from it, the threat response turned off. I didn't realize that at the time but now, with the practice of turning my focus elsewhere and learning not to compulsively check and monitor myself, I am able to manage my OCD. And, perhaps more importantly, when I can stop myself performing these checks and refocus my attentions elsewhere – I congratulate myself. I sit down and figure out how long it has been since the last time I was able to do it and I give myself praise for this achievement. Doing that has been really helpful.

Moving forward I have tried to keep my focus on the external because OCD thrives on the attention of thoughts, especially intrusive thoughts, and doing this has really helped me. I've still got a little way to go but I'm working with a CBT therapist as we speak and I've already made huge leaps in progress when it comes to the checking and compulsions. My anxiety has come down by 80 – 90% and I'm pleased to say that I'm living what is a normal life again.

Mairead

Chapter 11

In Sum

Featured Artist: @wholeheartedschoolcounselling

IF FEELINGS COULD TALK

🐻 by WholeHearted School Counseling

SADNESS might be telling me I need TO CRY

LONELINESS might be telling me I need CONNECTION

SHAME might be telling me I need SELF-COMPASSION

RESENTMENT might be telling me I need TO FORGIVE

EMPTINESS might be telling me I need TO DO SOMETHING CREATIVE

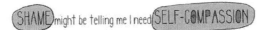

ANGER might be telling me I need TO CHECK-IN WITH MY BOUNDARIES

ANXIETY might be telling me I need TO BREATHE

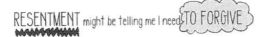

STRESS might be telling me I need TO TAKE IT ONE STEP AT A TIME

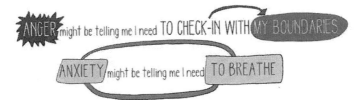

Thank you for taking the time to read this book. When we suffer with anxiety it can be difficult to stay focused and concentrate on absorbing all of this information but, you've done it!

In writing this book for you we've hoped to provide you with some reassurance and comfort by reducing your worries with a greater knowledge and understanding of anxiety. What we've come to learn is that anxiety does not mean that you are broken; on the contrary, your body is perfectly healthy and is doing its job almost *too well*. Armed with this information we hope to relieve you of the sense of continuous dread and use this as a stepping stone to realign with the non-anxious version of yourself.

Consider this a guide to understanding *your* anxiety. Anxiety is different for everyone so we have touched on the most typical presentations so that you can understand what it means for *you*. By combatting the negative thoughts, the 'what if's' and bringing you back to the present, the principles in this book will help you no matter how anxiety presents itself.

We're beyond happy to pass on our knowledge and expertise to you! Experience and education has us further along in our recovery but we have been in your shoes. Anxiety can feel like a huge weight that burdens us each and every day, but it can be easily dealt with when we have the know-how.

It is a pleasure for us to give you that know-how.

What we have here is an amalgamation of professional guidance and personal experience from people who actually *get it*. We are not citing this from a textbook, we are not robots, we have hearts, and have suffered just like you. We want this to give you hope.

There is a way out. Anyone can overcome their anxiety. It can feel like there is no end, but this does not have to be the case. We are here to guide you.

We're going to give you an overview of what we tackled throughout the book as a helpful reminder and a quick and easy way to find a specific section that you might benefit from re-reading.

Chapters 1 and 2 – What is anxiety?

You can start here when needing to conceptualise your anxiety. With anxiety being such a broad condition, it is worth distinguishing how it presents itself to you. Here is a brief overview of the common anxiety-related conditions discussed in this chapter:

Panic disorder or fear of panic – Becoming frightened of anxiety and panic attacks. This is rooted in avoidance for fear that something awful might happen.

Health Anxiety – This involves misinterpreting symptoms of anxiety as symptoms of something catastrophic. We might often find ourselves knocking on Dr Google's door seeking answers that often do not provide relief.

Social anxiety – A fear of how we are perceived by others. We can be crippled by how other people might view us which stops us from socialising or winds us up thinking about an event that is happening in three weeks' time.

Agoraphobia – A need to stay in what we consider a safe space. With agoraphobia outside is often deemed scary while inside is safe. We might think that *out there* something terrible might happen so it's best to stay inside.

Intrusive thoughts – These are unwanted thoughts that trigger anxiety. There are no boundaries with intrusive thoughts; they creep their way in without asking permission. They can be easily shaken off by your *Average Joe*, but the anxious person struggles to let it go. When the thoughts are particularly disturbing they can lead us to questioning who we are.

Obsessive compulsive disorder – OCD occurs when we believe that if we don't do X, Y and Z then something terrible is going to happen. We might believe that the survival of our family depends on us doing this action or behaviour. Typical behaviours include: cleaning, checking, picking or a mental routine of some sort.

Generalised anxiety disorder – This manifests as a constant worry over a variety of topics leaving us frequently feeling uneasy and on edge. Sometimes this includes worry about worrying!

Post-traumatic stress – This is experienced as a result of unprocessed trauma. When this is the case, we highly advise that you seek professional help.

Although there are more, these are the most common forms in which anxiety presents itself.

Chapter 3 – Why do we get the anxious response?

In this chapter we discussed the fear system built within us to keep us safe.

First we discussed **the amygdala,** found in the lizard brain. It is the oldest part of the brain but not the brightest as it can't always tell the difference between perceived danger and actual danger. It is the amygdala that makes us jump when we hear a car backfire or if someone jumps out of the dark. It is the conductor of fear, turning on and off in response to perceived threats.

In day-to-day situations we use both our **emotional brain** (where the amygdala can be found) and the **cognitive brain** (the thinking brain) to determine threat and the appropriate response. The two must work in tandem to respond and perceive things appropriately. However, with anxiety our emotional brain overruns the cognitive bran and denies us our rational thinking. For immediate danger we have no time to dilly dally, we need a rapid response. So, we cut out the middle man (the cognitive brain) and send sensory information straight to the amygdala. It can save our lives but is frustrating when unnecessary.

Adrenaline and cortisol – Here we discussed the feeling and purpose of adrenaline and cortisol in the threat response. As a quick reminder, adrenaline can be described as that 'whoosh' of energy that gets us moving! Whereas feeling on edge is likely a concoction of low level adrenaline and cortisol. It is the cortisol which keeps us in a state of hyper alert, prepared for any imminent danger.

Adrenaline can increase our heart rates, make us feel spaced out, nauseous, tense, or experience a sense of derealisation. It is an incredibly powerful hormone that can induce thoughts, feelings and physical changes.

The nervous system – Next we touched upon the autonomic nervous system (or just nervous system for ease). The nervous system is responsible for voluntary movement and internal processes that lie outside of our control.

In short, the *sympathetic nervous system* triggers fight, flight or freeze; triggering the adrenal glands (adrenaline) and altering the function of our vital organs. It handily adjusts our body's state to help manage stress every time we are in performance mode, stressed or under pressure. The sympathetic nervous system can be worn down with excessive anxiety, which results in feelings of exhaustion. However, when used correctly, it gets us through the hard times.

The *parasympathetic nervous system* is the restorative part of the nervous system. It activates during times of resting, sleeping, enjoyment and relief. This system lights up when we rest to help us regenerate, recoup and restore balance to the body's vital organs.

The role of stress in disordered anxiety – Remember the stress jug? With each experience of stress we add to the jug; everyday stress or trauma all contribute. We may be able to handle each little stressful experience as they come but, when they are not dealt with, the jug eventually overflows. This is when the *sympathetic nervous system* becomes exhausted and overused… cue anxiety disorder.

Overstressed and overworked *sympathetic nervous systems* trigger the amygdala, activating the threat response 'just in case'. In this case, the amygdala interprets our overflowing jug (excess stress) as danger. Built up stress over time puts strain on the sympathetic nervous system and tricks the amygdala into sensing danger. In turn we release adrenaline and cortisol hormones leaving us constantly feeling on edge without an understanding of why. This only contributes further to the *stress jug* until it is constantly overflowing. When this happens, the threat response never has the relief of turning off.

ANXIETY
might be a reminder to:

- Turn off the screen

- Check in and listen to your wise voice within

- Focus on what is within your control

- Treat yourself with gentle loving kindness

- Remember that not all thoughts are true

- Exercise (this helps to burn off the stress hormone cortisol)

- Deal with something you have been avoiding

- Get more sleep

- Take a few (or many) slow, deep & focused breaths

- Simply notice that you are feeling anxiety, without judgment

by WholeHearted School Counseling

Chapter 4 – The symptoms of anxiety

Let's have a quick recap and overview of the symptoms of anxiety.

Derealisation/depersonalisation – A feeling of unreality; detached from ourselves and our surroundings. This can also be described as an out-of-body experience and although it can feel uncomfortable, it is harmless.

This symptom can be caused by stress breathing and slow hyperventilation where we intake more oxygen than we need and do not exhale enough carbon dioxide. Alternatively, when in fight or flight, this response restricts blood flow to the brain to distribute more blood to major muscle groups helping us fight or flee if necessary. This can also lead us to feeling spaced out.

Hyperventilating – This consists of shallow and restricted breathing in the form of short, sharp intakes of breath. This breathing pattern can seemingly come out of nowhere but may cause an anxious person to panic. In turn, this continues the quick and shallow breathing causing further hyperventilation and panic. It can also be initiated from pent up tension in the upper body which affects the ability of the diaphragm to function effectively. Tension in these areas can lead to breathlessness which can trigger worry and panic in an anxiety sufferer.

Struggling to catch breath – Our bodies are so good at self-regulation that they can stop us inhaling further when we have *too much oxygen*! By preventing us from taking in more oxygen than we need, we can feel as though we cannot catch our breath or fill our lungs. This contributes to further panic in an anxiety sufferer.

Heart Palpitations – Our heartbeat increases due to the adrenaline and cortisol released when we feel anxious. It is a normal and natural response to these hormones but can leave us fearing that something else is wrong.

Digestive system problems – The symptoms of anxiety can mimic symptoms of IBS. When anxious, the threat response is our top priority and digestion comes second. We press pause on the digestive tract while we place our energy elsewhere in the body ready for when we need to engage the fight or flight response. It does this to keep us safe but the effects of this can include bloating, diarrhoea, stomach cramps and other related symptoms.

Chest pain – chest pain often occurs due to muscle tension and posture. Muscles contract as we engage the threat response, ready to flee and save ourselves. When we relax, we can feel this chest pain which causes panic, especially when coupled with heart palpitations, as we can be left feeling as though we might be experiencing a panic attack. If you have any concerns, you must check with a doctor to make sure.

Sweating/Perspiration – When in fight or flight mode we release adrenaline which activates our sweat glands. For an anxious person, hypersensitivity makes us hyper aware of our perspiration which can lead to excessive sweating. Sweating is part of everyday life and not limited to anxiety disorders but someone with anxiety focuses on how much they are sweating which can lead them to sweat even more.

Problems with sleep – The sleep/anxiety feedback loop can be difficult for a lot of people. Anxiety can *cause* lack of or broken sleep which in turn *raises* our anxiety levels. As much as one third of the adult population reports difficulty sleeping so as we said, you are not alone! Insomnia and nightmares are listed as common symptoms in general anxiety disorder. Sleep problems impact how we function emotionally, mentally and physically. Treating one often helps the other but treating both is the best recipe for success.

Difficulty concentrating – This is when we find ourselves hyper focusing on a thought that distracts us from everything else in life. When stuck with this thought in our head it can be hard to concentrate on anything else. 'Lack of concentrating' is misleading because the opposite is in fact true. You are concentrating except you are laser focused on the wrong things, like the anxiety you feel.

Chapter 5 – Anxiety is a threat response

In this chapter we looked at the necessity to describe anxiety as the threat response. Here are the key takeaway points discussed:

Excessive anxiety is a problem when the threat response misfires when we don't want it to. You are not broken. Anxious thoughts and vivid imaginations are signs of intelligence. That's right, you smart cookie. It becomes a problem when we begin to imagine the worst case scenarios in situations where we are otherwise safe. The threat response becomes triggered by even the most minute detail, prompting the rationalisation process when it simply isn't needed.

Overcoming anxiety is all about *turning off the threat response*. It sounds so simple, and it could be. When there is no immediate danger that requires us to fight, run or freeze, we need to train our brains to flick the switch and turn the threat response off.

We cannot talk to the amygdala and persuade it to calm down or take a chill pill. Talking doesn't work, we need to *show it*. We show it by using our senses and facing our fears. When we face the fear and *show* the threat response that we aren't in danger, and don't require its assistance, we can begin to function and live our normal lives again.

The threat response is necessary. It kept our ancestors alive and remains an integral asset in keeping us free from harm. Remaining on high alert allows us to see the danger coming and quicker engage with adrenaline which gets us out of there! However, in everyday life we can become easily confused. We still need the threat response because there will be situations where we might need to take off and protect ourselves, but this rarely happens in modern day life. We simply must show the amygdala that we are not in danger and *turn the threat response off.*

Chapter 6 – Exposure done right

In chapter 6 we explained the ins and outs of exposure therapy and how to do it right! Here are the key points discussed:

Jumping back to the previous chapter, we discussed the necessity for *showing* the amygdala that we are safe, pleading with it simply will not do. This is where *exposure therapy* comes into play. The more we expose ourselves to these perceived 'dangerous' situations the more we can show the brain that actually, we're quite safe and we can turn the threat response off.

But there are effective and ineffective ways to practice exposure therapy. White-knuckling your way through and forcing yourself into situations that you don't want to be in, you guessed it… doesn't work! We must practice exposure therapy with the knowledge of *why* we are doing it and a *reassurance* that we are safe.

Secondary fear – Secondary fear is also known as a *phobia*; this phobia being a fear of our own anxious response. Everyone experiences anxiety to some degree. However, when it becomes excessive we often develop a secondary fear which is a fear of anxiety itself. With exposure therapy we *redefine our relationship* with our fear response. By doing this we are not only able to turn off the threat response but conquer this secondary fear (phobia) at the same time by practising the act of just *being with it* when it arises.

Safety behaviours – Absolute avoidance and micro-avoidance

Safety behaviours are seemingly useful in reducing anxiety in the short term but become a problem as they encourage anxiety in the long term. They stop us facing our fears head on for the comfort of the here and now, yet contribute to further anxiety and discomfort in the future. Remember our stress jug? Yeah, you get it.

Two categories we looked at:

1. **Absolute avoidance** – It does what it says on the tin. We categorically avoid things for fear of how they will make us feel. Recovery begins with challenging absolute avoidance so we can start showing the threat response that we are in fact safe in these situations.

2. **Micro-avoidance** – This is where 'white-knuckling' our way through an experience might come into play. We're trying to be brave enough to do something we've been avoiding but still in need of some form of false comfort to get us through. Ultimately, we aren't able to overcome the fear because we relied upon safety items, safe people or being aware of all the exits to get us through. By doing this, we aren't fully sitting with the fear and so we don't give ourselves the credit for making it through either; the credit is awarded to these false comforts. We must remove these false comforts and fully immerse ourselves in the discomfort to show the amygdala that we are in fact safe.

Graded exposure vs flooding – Next, we spoke about graded exposure and flooding. Graded exposure means gradually upping the exposure to the fear we wish to overcome. We progressively take one step closer to the fear over time so that we don't become overwhelmed by discomfort. We increase the exposure until the amygdala comes to realise that it is safe in this situation.

Flooding, however, is diving straight into the deep end and exposing ourselves to the most difficult stimuli straight away. It sounds scary, but it works just as effectively as graded exposure. If you're feeling eager to jump straight in, then have it! Most choose graded exposure to begin with as clients tend to feel more comfortable with taking small steps and it also makes it feel achievable.

Two types of exposure in CBT - In vivo vs imaginal and internal vs external.

Remember, **in vivo** refers to *real-world exposure* to the feared stimuli. For example, if we had a fear of dogs, we could easily find a willing pup to help us with exposure therapy. However some exposure is not possible, such as with PTSD clients or survivors of domestic abuse. In this case we use **imaginal exposure** where we can vividly describe and imagine a situation using all of our senses. This works best with a trained therapist!

When looking at **internal vs external** we are discussing where we receive our *exposure cues. External cues* can include things like a fear of heights, fear of spiders or fear of balloons whereas *internal cues* are when we respond to inner sensations, fears and worries. A lot of anxiety is internal and so a CBT technique called *interoceptive exposure* is helpful for people who are frightened of their own anxious sensations. With internal cues we might induce worrisome thoughts, increase our heart rate by running on the spot, or revisit painful memories. We try to bring about the same feelings induced by anxiety in order to expose ourselves to them and desensitise.

Exposure if we are just anxious at home is just as necessary. The best way to integrate exposure therapy in day to day life is to **continue on with your day as if the anxiety is not present.** By doing what we would usually do, regardless of our anxiety levels, we can begin to train the amygdala to turn the threat response off as we are showing it that it is safe to do so.

Chapter 7 - Cultivating a new attitude

Throughout chapter 7 we reinforce the necessity for cultivating a different attitude toward anxiety. As Josh said, we cannot challenge anxiety if we are being critical of ourselves, there is absolutely no point. By utilising the knowledge in books like this we can develop a stronger understanding for what exactly it is that we are dealing with, and with this knowledge, we can overcome it effectively. Yet this all must begin with a new attitude.

Remember to **see anxiety as a spectrum not binary.** Anxiety is not black and white, on or off. There are levels, like a ten-tiered sponge cake. It is helpful to rate your anxiety on a scale of 1 to 10 in order to gain some perspective and regain some control. By using this technique you can more greatly understand your own anxiety levels which in turn will make them easier to manage.

Use **cognitive reframing** to take an original belief and view it from a positive perspective. The original belief remains but we have reframed it in a way that it becomes beneficial to us. For example, "What if I get scared at the conference and freeze in front of everyone?" becomes "The conference is the perfect opportunity for me to practise tolerating my anxiety". We still acknowledge that the situation is fear inducing but we shift how we approach the situation to one that is helpful to us.

This brought us ever so neatly to **wilful tolerance**. Remember the 'white-knuckling' that we spoke of earlier, well we ideally want to avoid this. Wilful tolerance means approaching scary situations *willingly,* appreciating that it is ok to be scared and that it will likely be uncomfortable but ultimately we know that there isn't any real danger. This is how we rewire our brains – we must remind ourselves that we want to *turn off the threat response* and that we are willing to experience this temporary discomfort to do so.

Practise wilful tolerance with self-compassion. Be kind to yourself and focus on the positives in each experience. You aren't expected to master this straight away, so give yourself credit for the little victories.

Inner dialogue learned from our youth concluded chapter 7. This is where we looked at how our anxiety is influenced by the beliefs we learn as a child. We derive meaning from the words and behaviours of those around us at a time where are brains are forming, we infer meaning from these words and behaviours that contribute to our inner dialogue. When we catch our inner dialogue criticising us about our anxiety, we must ask ourselves, "What am I absorbing?" and "Where have I learned this from?"

WHAT TO TELL MYSELF WHEN I'M FEELING DISCOURAGED

by WholeHearted School Counseling

1. This is tough. But so am I.

2. I may not be able to control this situation. But I am in charge of how I respond.

3. I haven't figured this out...yet.

4. This challenge is here to teach me something.

5. All I need to do is take it one step at a time. Breathe. And do the next right thing.

Chapter 8 - How to deal with anxiety attacks

Chapter 8 looks over a few techniques that we really love that have helped both of us tolerate our anxiety attacks. Let's quickly summarise what we discussed in this chapter:

The first technique covered utilised the cognitive reframing technique. Try reframing it as an **adrenaline rush, not a panic attack**. Quite frankly, it sounds less scary and is in fact more accurate.

Neuroception helps us better understand the involuntary nervous system which looks at two major components: the sympathetic nervous system and the parasympathetic nervous system. The sympathetic nervous system is responsible for engaging the fight, flight or freeze response whereas the parasympathetic nervous system is responsible for rest, relaxation and digestion. We want these two systems to work in harmony and forever return to a state of balance.

When experiencing a panic attack, it is helpful and reassuring to understand how these two systems are working. By acknowledging that our sympathetic nervous system is overworked and over stressed, in need of emptying the stress jug, it can make it easier to tolerate a panic attack.

Stop trying to resist and fix reinforced the notion that the best thing we can do during an anxious episode is acknowledge that this is the *threat response*. The more we try to resist and fight these feelings the greater the chance that we will make our anxiety worse. The best thing to do is *to continue with what you were doing*, carry on with your day and, utilise the knowledge you have of what is going on in your body to comfort you. This will show the threat response that you are safe and that it is not needed.

Allow the body to regulate itself explains how our bodies know exactly what to do in order to bring us back to balance. The body will always restore order and so trusting your body to what it does best is perhaps the best thing we can do during an anxiety attack. Bringing us back to a state of balance and equilibrium is what the body excels at. So, whatever the situation or intensity of your anxiety, even when *you* don't know what to do, the body *does*. It will restore balance between the sympathetic and parasympathetic nervous systems.

However, if you are experiencing intense feelings of anxiety then you can jump back to chapter 8 where, in this last section, we discuss two different **grounding techniques** and one **breathing technique** which can help you tolerate the anxiety attack.

Note: these are not quick fixes! They will simply help you cope until the body does its work.

Chapter 9 - Handpicked tips and tricks!

This covered the following sections:

- Scale your anxiety

- Stop monitoring and score points

- Engage the present

- Less doing, more being

- The body fixes itself

- The alarm analogy

- Parasympathetic activities

- Making something else the centre of your life.

This is the chapter you want to jump back to for our favourite and most recommended practices for helping you on your recovery journey. Once you've read the rest of the book and feel comfortable with your new understanding of anxiety as the *threat response*, we encourage you to go through this chapter a handful of times. Greater understanding of the biological necessity for anxiety is extremely helpful, implement this in your day-to-day life with the tips and tricks in chapter 9 and see what happens!

Chapter 10 – Success Stories

Here we shared with you some success stories from our community. Ultimately, nothing is more encouraging than knowing that someone else has been through the same struggle as you and managed to come out the other side. The journey of recovery is different for everyone however; hearing the stories of others can encourage us and make us feel less alone. You are not alone. Find comfort in our community and solidarity in our struggles and victories. We've been there and we know how it feels, that is why we have written this book. So you can feel like there is a way out, that you can overcome your anxiety, and that there are people out there who know exactly how you feel and can support you.

We truly hope that this book has been helpful in giving you greater insight and understanding of anxiety. The more we know the better equipped we are to handle this condition and, if you're reading this book, you're certainly on your way to living a non-anxious life. Implement the techniques discussed and see the difference they can make. These are all exercises that we have both used in our own anxiety recoveries so they have not been regurgitated from a textbook; they have been tried and tested.

We wish you the best of luck in your recovery and, if you do know of anyone who would benefit from reading this book then please do pass it on! The more people we can help, the better.

Manufactured by Amazon.ca
Bolton, ON

19097957R00101